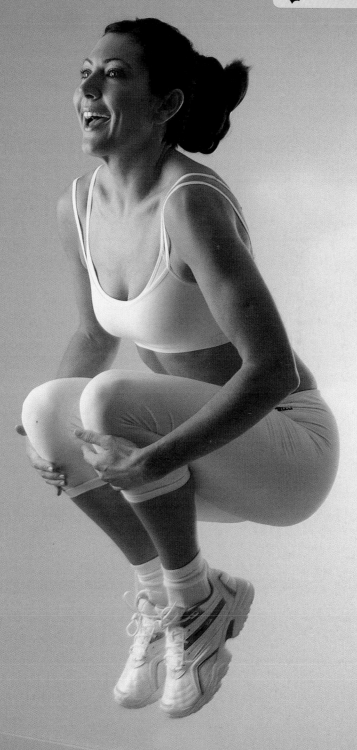

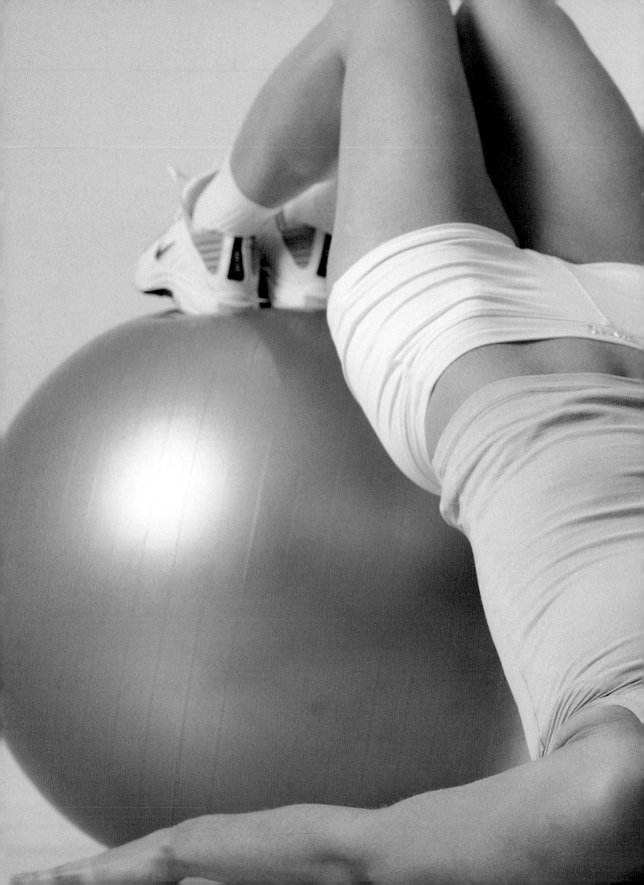

Matt Roberts

THE PHA
WORKOUT

halve your workout time
the revolutionary new system

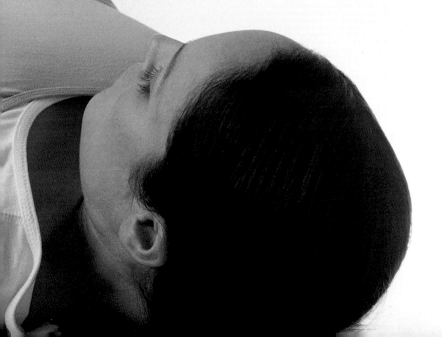

LONDON, NEW YORK, MELBOURNE,
MUNICH and DELHI

Project Editor Susannah Steel
Project Art Editor Ruth Hope
Managing Editor Stephanie Farrow
Managing Art Editor Marianne Markham
Art Director Carole Ash
Publishing Manager Gillian Roberts
Publishing Director Mary-Clare Jerram
DTP Designer Sonia Charbonnier
Production Controller Shane Higgins
Photographer John Davis

First published in the Great Britain in 2005
by Dorling Kindersley Limited
80 Strand, London WC2R 0RL
A Penguin Company

**Always consult your doctor before starting
a fitness programme if you have any
health concerns.**

Every effort has been made to ensure that the
information in this book is accurate. However, neither
the publisher, nor the author, nor anyone else involved
in the preparation of this book are engaged in
rendering professional advice or services to the
individual reader.

A CIP catalogue record for this book is available
from the British Library.

ISBN 1 4053 0326 3

Colour reproduction by GRB, Italy
Printed and bound by Star Standard, Singapore

Discover more at
www.dk.com

contents

author's introduction

Part of the job of being a personal trainer is about "selling the dream", and then having the ability to back this up and teach people the practical skills they need to fulfil this dream. And for many of us, the dream is simply a desire to fit a successful workout regime into our busy lifestyles.

Whilst wishing to give people the chance to fulfil their dreams in as short a time as possible, I don't want to give the impression that exercising for just eight minutes a day, or one hour per week, or even at your office desk, would actually be effective. Any fitness programmes that promise you will change your shape or lose weight – or, indeed, pretty much any other health target – in such tiny periods of time are just blatant lies.

I can, however, make a very bold promise, and be sure that it holds true. I can teach you how to halve your workout time. The reason I can make this promise, and be certain of its success, is that the technique I will show you in this book is one that focuses on eliminating the weaknesses from your current, conventional workout regime. Whilst you won't learn any "new" exercises as such, the major change to your routine will be in the method of exercising that I will push you through: PHA training.

Peripheral Heart Action (PHA) is a dynamic change to your routine that will lift your current fitness level to new and unexpected heights, and give you the opportunity to reach your goals without having to commit to excessive hours of additional training.

This is the promise that I stand by, and I believe it is the solution that many people search for and never find in trying to achieve their personal goals.

The PHA technique that I will show you is one that has never, to my knowledge, been documented and researched in the ways that I have done with my clients and for this book. Since I started my company, my team of trainers has accumulated more than 100,000 hours of "hands on" personal training with clients. It is this resource of information that has given me incredible access to the real results of how various exercise techniques benefit people in different ways. What I know from our combined experience is that PHA training produces phenomenal results for a variety of different fitness goals. At present, it is probably the most under-utilized technique in the exercise industry. In writing this book, I want to introduce you to the method that I think will revolutionize your workouts.

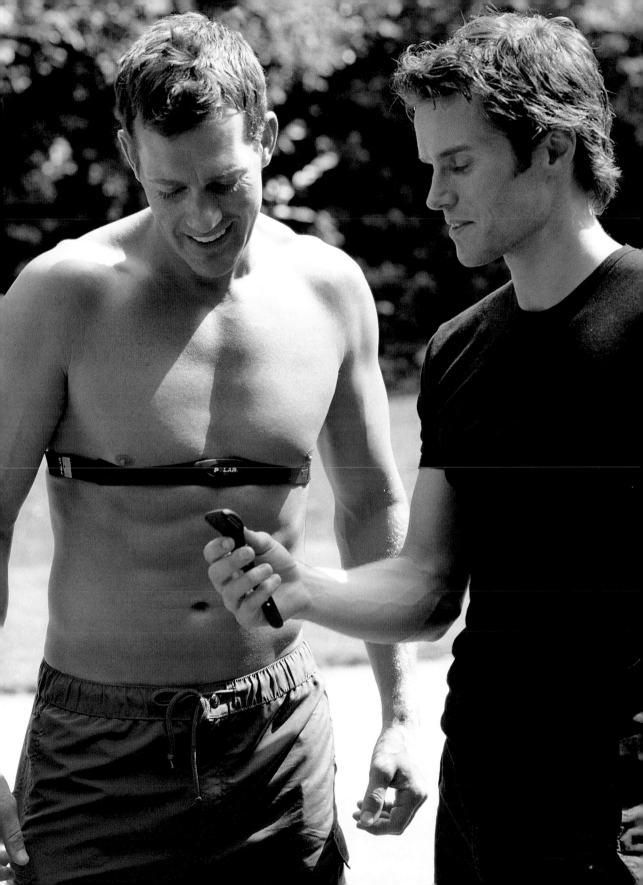

about PHA

Peripheral Heart Action (PHA) training is a dynamic way of exercising using controlled resistance training with weights – which increases the tone and strength of your muscles – in a way that makes your heart pump faster, like aerobic exercise. What this means is that PHA training can give you all the benefits of these two different types of workout in the time it takes to do just one, with great results.

Why use PHA training?

The quickest way for most people to become fitter is to continuously work the heart and lungs to their maximum limit. PHA training achieves this with a time-efficient workout sequence that alternates between upper and lower body muscles (*see* muscle groups, *p. 11*) with every exercise. This varies from the conventional "stop/start" approach to resistance training, in which exercises for one muscle group at a time are performed back-to-back, with a rest in between each set.

I've been using the PHA training system with clients who want to lose weight and reduce their overall body fat, and they've experienced very rapid results. I've also been able to focus my clients' attention into shorter, more intensive periods of time than conventional exercise allows.

The PHA technique has also been used very effectively with athletes, footballers, and, most significantly, triathletes, who benefit enormously from the ongoing shifts in workload between the upper and lower body. This "consistent intensity" approach to training suits the demands of these team sports players and endurance athletes very well: it encourages their fitness to be continually challenged while, at the same time, not

overloading any one particular area of the body, which could result in muscle injury. As a user of PHA training myself, I can assure you that you will stimulate as many muscle fibres as possible without incurring muscle soreness or damage: by varying the muscle groups you use for every exercise, the body has time to recover adequately. This ensures that your performance levels remain high and your muscles function efficiently.

The PHA system

So how does PHA combine the all benefits of two separate conventional fitness programmes? If the intention of working out was purely to maintain a high working heart rate, aerobic training would be the most obvious way of achieving that goal. However, we now know that people who only do aerobic training achieve less in their workouts than those people who combine resistance and aerobic training. Likewise, resistance training doesn't generally burn enough energy during a workout. Instead, it builds muscle mass, which does have the desirable effect of increasing the metabolic rate by stimulating muscles to use energy more readily.

PHA training blends aerobic and resistance training into one system that allows for greater energy-burning levels during a training session, and long-term energy-burning effects from a raised metabolic rate.

Raising your metabolic rate

It is common for people who exercise hard to feel hot and "racing" for several hours after a workout, which is a visible sign of a raised metabolic rate. After-burn, the result of a high metabolism, is now

PHA **burns fat** and **tones muscle** by working the **upper** and **lower** body **alternately** using **resistance training**

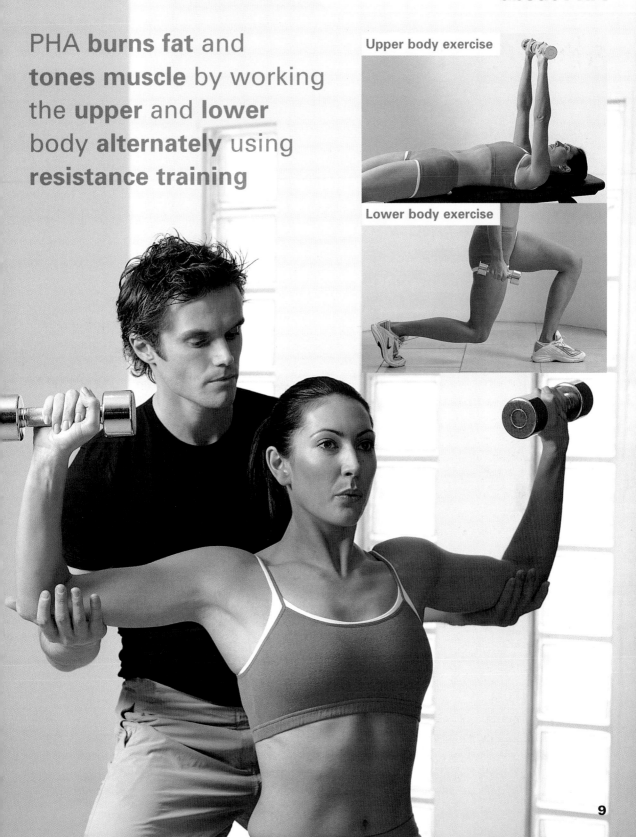

Upper body exercise

Lower body exercise

your heart rate during a workout

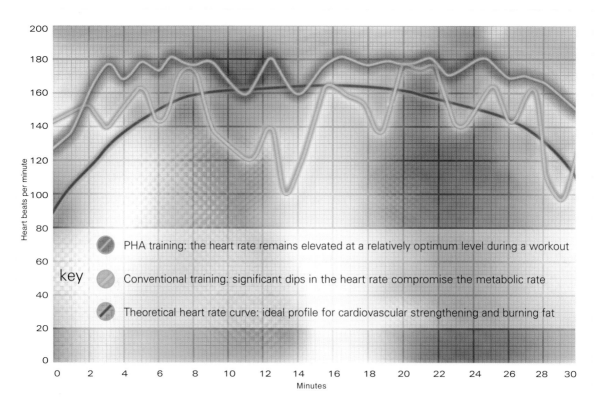

key
- PHA training: the heart rate remains elevated at a relatively optimum level during a workout
- Conventional training: significant dips in the heart rate compromise the metabolic rate
- Theoretical heart rate curve: ideal profile for cardiovascular strengthening and burning fat

known to be a fundamental part of long-term fat loss, and it is essential for the maintenance of a lean body. Thus, a high metabolic rate is one of the most valuable and effective ways of losing weight.

If you look at statistical evidence charting the heart rate of someone on a conventional fitness programme and someone on one of my PHA workouts (*see chart, above*), you can see why the PHA technique improves the metabolic rate so effectively and establishes good after-burn. By alternately working upper and lower muscle groups (*see right*) using intensive PHA-based resistance exercises, you should be able to raise your heart rate (in orange, *above*) to roughly 85 per cent of your maximum heart rate (*p.19*). This enables you to burn fat and reach appropriate muscle overload (when muscles are challenged and become stronger).

Lost workload

When you compare the profile of an average 30-year-old person's conventional resistance training session (in green, *above*) against the elevated heart rate achieved on the PHA workout, you'll see that the conventional workout reveals significant dips in heart rate levels throughout the exercise period. Such inconsistency compromises the potential effectiveness of the workout itself. This variable rate is a result of the stop/start approach of conventional resistance training, which prevents your heart rate from maintaining a sufficiently high level to keep burning calories. Your heart rate commonly falls by 15–20 per cent within a minute of stopping exercise and this drop-off rate is, in effect, lost workload on your body. It is this aspect that can be altered by using the PHA system.

muscle groups

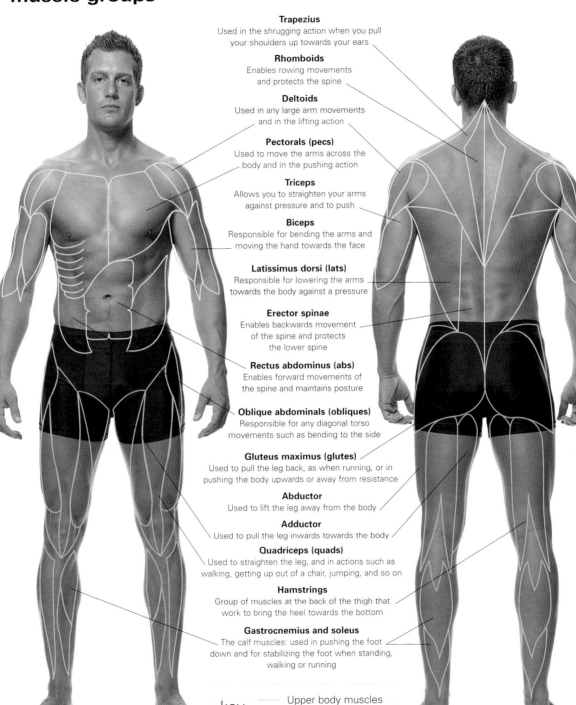

Trapezius
Used in the shrugging action when you pull your shoulders up towards your ears

Rhomboids
Enables rowing movements and protects the spine

Deltoids
Used in any large arm movements and in the lifting action

Pectorals (pecs)
Used to move the arms across the body and in the pushing action

Triceps
Allows you to straighten your arms against pressure and to push

Biceps
Responsible for bending the arms and moving the hand towards the face

Latissimus dorsi (lats)
Responsible for lowering the arms towards the body against a pressure

Erector spinae
Enables backwards movement of the spine and protects the lower spine

Rectus abdominus (abs)
Enables forward movements of the spine and maintains posture

Oblique abdominals (obliques)
Responsible for any diagonal torso movements such as bending to the side

Gluteus maximus (glutes)
Used to pull the leg back, as when running, or in pushing the body upwards or away from resistance

Abductor
Used to lift the leg away from the body

Adductor
Used to pull the leg inwards towards the body

Quadriceps (quads)
Used to straighten the leg, and in actions such as walking, getting up out of a chair, jumping, and so on

Hamstrings
Group of muscles at the back of the thigh that work to bring the heel towards the bottom

Gastrocnemius and soleus
The calf muscles: used in pushing the foot down and for stabilizing the foot when standing, walking or running

key
Upper body muscles
Lower body muscles

introduction

You can expect to burn up to 10 per cent more calories a day on a PHA programme, even when going about your daily business. The ongoing effects of this training system have such a pronounced boosting effect on your body that the benefits can continue for up to 36 hours in a moderate capacity. When you add on the extra calories burnt during your four workouts each week, plus the after-burn boost you get in those initial post-exercise hours, you'll find that there is an enormous amount of extra potential for burning calories.

Maximum effort, minimum time

The fact that PHA can also halve your workout time is based on the premise that we'll reduce your training "dead time" to a minimum by ensuring that you'll work the body continuously: as the upper body muscles work, the lower body rests, then you'll swap to work the lower body, and the cycle continues. The PHA technique focuses on using major muscle groups for most exercises, and since these muscle groups require the greatest amount of blood flow to them, they are, therefore,

burning the greatest number of calories possible. As blood is shunted up and down the body to these muscles, your metabolic rate rises significantly, your heart and lung functioning is overloaded, and your muscle stimulation is heightened.

The four PHA programmes

Normally, a fitness regime that reduces fat levels would take 40–45 minutes to complete, but on the PHA Fat loss programme you'll work at high intensity for only 20 minutes at a time, with great results. Likewise, creating muscle tone usually necessitates 45–60 minutes of work per session, but on the Muscle-sculpting plan it takes just 30 minutes. The PHA Bulking up programme, which is a special sequence of upper and lower body exercises designed to build muscle mass and strength, takes a mere 40 minutes to complete. The weights that you'll be using for these three PHA programmes are self-adjusting: start with light weights, and when the number of reps you perform begins to feel easy, increase the weight by approximately 10 per cent on your next workout.

The workouts

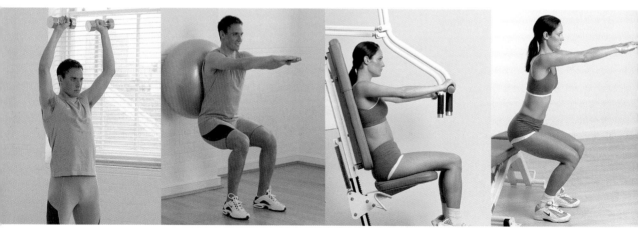

workout 1 fat loss

workout 2 muscle-sculpting

Finally, the 45-minute Endurance plan will give you greater stamina and muscular endurance using slightly lighter weights and more aerobic speed.

Perform these workouts four times a week, for a minimum of six weeks, to reap the benefits. You needn't limit yourself to just one workout either: the programmes complement each other (*see Questions & Answers, pp.44–45, 76–77, 122–23, 152–53*), and are suitable for both men and women. Once you've seen good results on one programme, re-assess your goals and try another workout to improve other aspects of your fitness. The Fat loss plan can be done at home, and the others are gym-based, but I've also included alternative travel workouts so that you can keep training whenever you are away from home or the gym.

The optimum way to exercise

All these promises from one fitness system are, for many of us, the "Holy Grail". Our busy lifestyles dictate that we must squeeze our activities into small amounts of time. Does this mean that if we had more time, we might do things differently? While there are some fitness goals that could be achieved using a less time-efficient approach, such as building muscle, all other fitness goals are most effectively met using the PHA system. This method is one that I now use most frequently with the majority of my clients who have struggled to

The **PHA system** truly suits **anyone** when used **correctly**

achieve their fitness goals before seeing me. If I want to give a client a real blitz before their film role or music video, I use the PHA technique to reduce excess water retention and create tone over the entire body. If I want to take a premiership footballer to a higher level of fitness, this technique forms the bedrock of all the resistance training that we do. The PHA system truly suits anyone when used in the correct way.

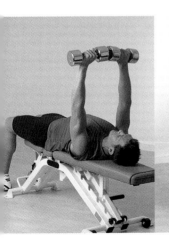
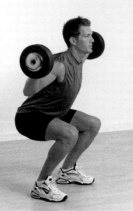
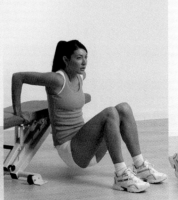
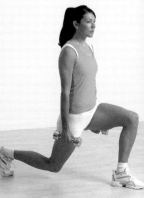

workout 3 bulking up

workout 4 endurance

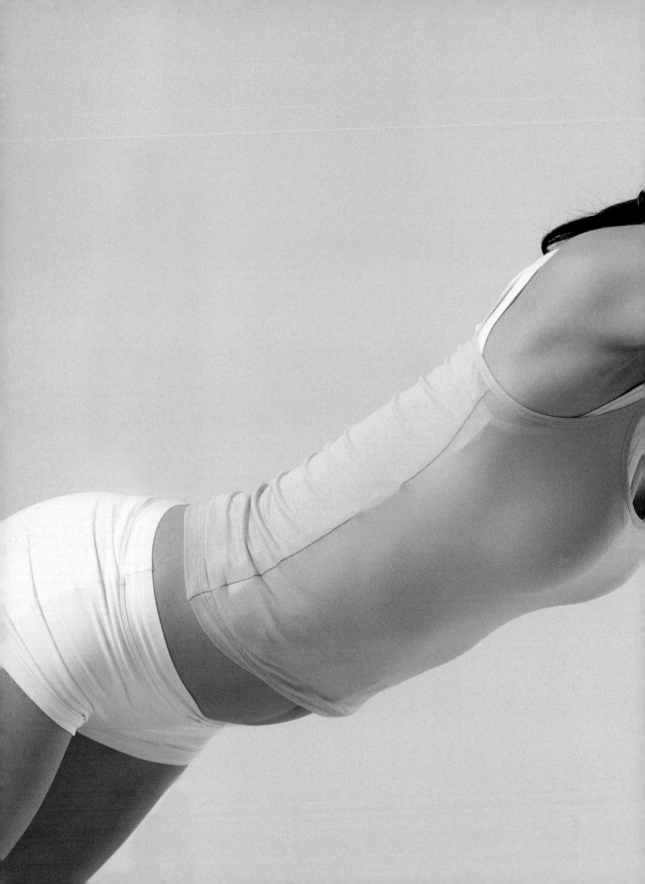

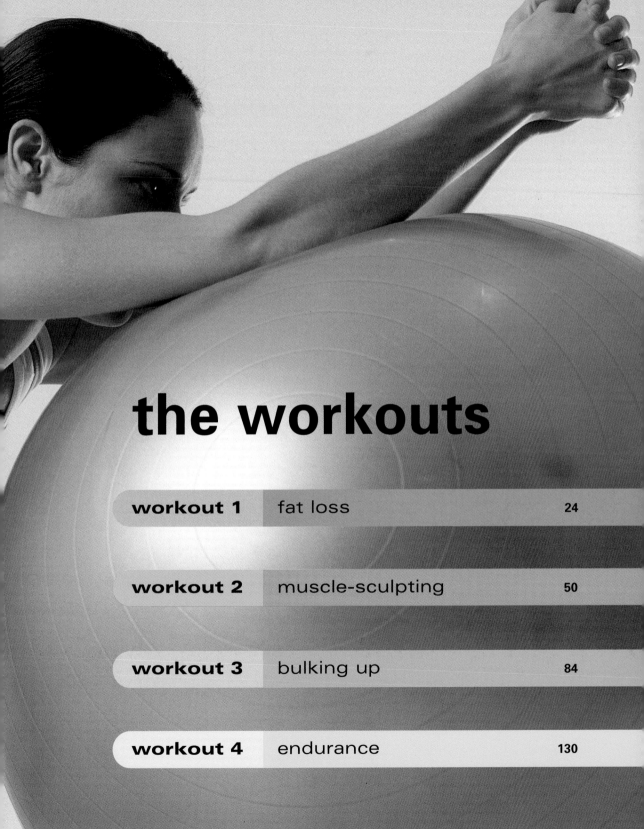

the workouts

warming up

The warm-up period is an essential precursor to any workout. This is the preparation time that your body needs in order to prevent any injury or discomfort during the higher intensity of effort required in the main PHA workout.

Prior to exercise, your body is probably working at a fairly comfortable, sedate pace. At this level, the body can control muscles, ligaments, tendons, vital organs, and also bones, without strain. Once you start exercising, however, these areas of the body

1 select an aerobic warm-up exercise

Warm up the major muscle groups in your body for a minimum of six minutes. Choose your preferred form of aerobic exercise – such as rowing, running, walking, stair-climbing, or using a cross-trainer. Start slowly and give yourself time to get into your stride to wake your muscles up properly.

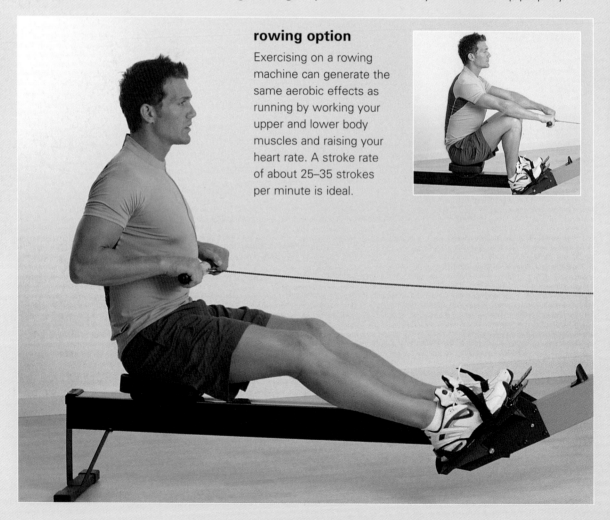

rowing option

Exercising on a rowing machine can generate the same aerobic effects as running by working your upper and lower body muscles and raising your heart rate. A stroke rate of about 25–35 strokes per minute is ideal.

must work much harder, and so they are put under much greater stress. An effective warm-up period of just six to nine minutes helps to prepare the body for high-impact exercise. Extra blood is gradually delivered to the muscles to fuel them with oxygen for the work ahead, while vital lubricators in the body build up in the high-stress areas around the joints and skeletal hinge areas.

Choose your warm-up

It's up to you how you choose to warm up before a workout. In a gym environment, try exercise machines such as a cross-trainer or rowing machine, which effectively warm up the muscles in both the upper and lower body. If you are exercising at home, I would recommend five to six minutes of stair-climbing or a six- to eight-minute

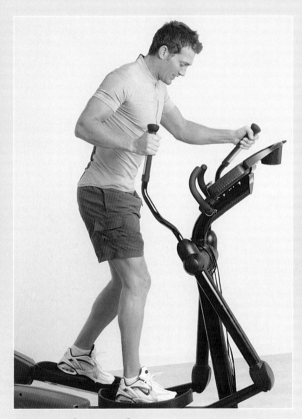

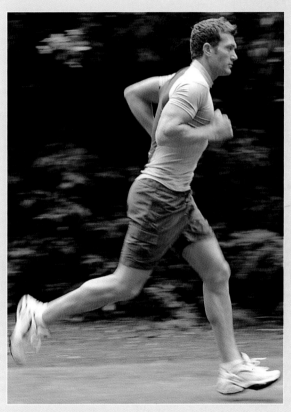

cross-trainer option

This piece of equipment, also known as an elliptical motion machine, is an effective alternative to a treadmill or cross-country skier machine, and it works a wider range of lower body muscles evenly. It also takes the impact out of the action of running, so avoiding the risk of knee injury. Remember to work your arms hard, as it's easy to forget them while powering away with your legs.

running option

Aerobic exercise such as running is essential to any fitness programme, and is an ideal way to warm the body up before a workout. Run for six to nine minutes and you'll warm up your muscles and get your circulation going; run for 30 to 40 minutes and you'll raise your heart rate to an optimum level that will, in turn, improve your body metabolism and maximize the effectiveness of your PHA workout.

fast-paced walk to raise the pulse rate. If you go for a run outdoors, you can, if you wish, spend up to half an hour running to achieve a good working heart rate (*below right*). In fact, 30 minutes of any aerobic sport in conjunction with PHA training is a good thing: run or row three to four times a week if you want to reap the maximum benefits from your PHA programme.

Take it by degrees

Allow your body to build itself up by degrees as you warm up. Take a few minutes to accelerate up to a comfortable pace, gradually making your movements bigger as you do so. Big muscle groups – the quads, hamstrings, chest, and back – are your major "motors" for the body when you're working out, and are responsible for increasing the

② stretch your upper body muscles

By the time you've spent six minutes or more working aerobically, you should have warmed up all the major muscle groups in your body. Then perform this short sequence of stretches to ensure that you also warm up your upper body muscles and get movement into your spine.

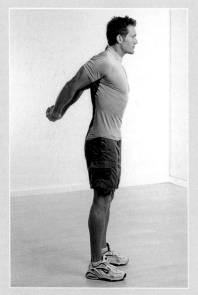

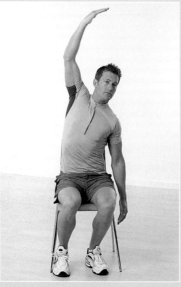

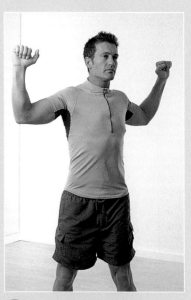

① chest stretch

A gentle stretch for the chest and shoulder muscles. Don't tilt forwards as you raise your hands.

- Stand upright with feet hip-width apart
- Clasp hands behind back
- Straighten arms
- Raise hands up
- Hold for 15–20 seconds

② arm reachover

This action stretches your lats and gets movement into your spine. Hold your hips square and still, and don't lean sideways as you stretch. Repeat on both sides.

- Sit upright and raise your arm above your head
- Pull your shoulder and upper body away from your hips
- Hold for 15–20 seconds

③ spinal rotation

This stretch also loosens your spine and warms up your oblique muscles. Hold your torso still.

- Stand upright with feet hip-width apart
- Keep hips in line with your knees and toes
- Raise elbows to shoulder-height and rotate slowly from side to side for 20 seconds

blood demand around the body, so you must warm up these muscles effectively. Once you've done this, do the three upper body stretches (*below left*).

Elevating your heart rate

One of the most important areas to keep track of in a PHA workout is your heart rate. We are trying to keep your heart rate elevated to give it an element of aerobic training, and your warm-up should raise your heart rate sufficiently for this. Take your pulse manually or check your heart rate monitor (*p.158*) at the end of the warm-up, then check to see if your heart rate is within your "optimum training zone" (*see chart, below*). Aim to keep your heart rate consistently at 75–85 per cent of your maximum heart rate (MHR) during the workout.

③ calculate your % maximum heart rate (MHR)

To be certain that you are working at the correct percentage of your maximum heart rate, work out your heart beats per minute (BPM), then check against the relevant age group (*see chart, below*) to see if your heart rate is within your optimum training zone of 75–85%MHR.

You can also calculate your optimum training heart rate by assuming that your MHR is 220 at birth, and then deleting your age from that figure. So, for example, if you are 30 years old, your MHR is 190PBPM and your optimum training heart rate is therefore 144–163BPM.

The workouts included in this book are designed to be performed intensively within certain time limits in order to raise your heart rate to its optimum training zone. If you are aged 65 or over, or if you have a medical condition, you should consult a doctor before you begin a PHA programme.

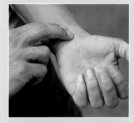 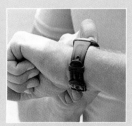

check your BPM

Take your pulse manually (*above left*), or use a heart rate monitor chest strap and watch (*above right*), which is specially designed to do the job. To feel for your pulse at your wrist, follow the line of your thumb, and then place two fingers just below your wrist joint. Count for 15 seconds, then multiply by four to get a beats per minute (BPM) figure.

rate of exertion

As a general guideline, at 65–75%MHR you will be aware of your breathing, but still able to hold a conversation; at 80%MHR you will be breathing heavily and just able to hold a conversation; and at 85%MHR you will be sweating and find it difficult to hold a conversation.

optimum training zone					
age	65%MHR	70%MHR	75%MHR	80%MHR	85%MHR
18–25	130	139	149	159	169
26–30	127	134	144	153	163
31–36	124	130	140	149	158
37–42	120	126	135	144	153
43–50	116	121	129	138	147
51–58	112	116	124	133	141
59–65	108	110	118	126	134
66+	104	106	114	121	129

cooling down

Taking the time to stretch your muscles at the end of every workout is essential. If you don't stretch effectively after you've finished a workout session, you'll inhibit the flexibility and mobility of your body, and risk injury or muscle damage.

Conditioning your muscles

The warm-up was your first chance to prevent any potential damage caused by the constant activity required of a PHA workout. Remember that the PHA technique raises the intensity of your

stretching sequence

This 10-minute stretching sequence will help to alleviate any muscle soreness or discomfort in your muscles after you've finished a workout.

Don't rush through the stretches: aim to spend a minimum of 15 seconds stretching each muscle. Hold the pose for longer to get a deeper stretch.

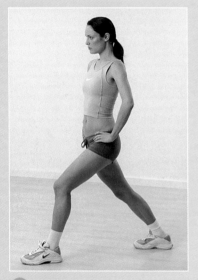 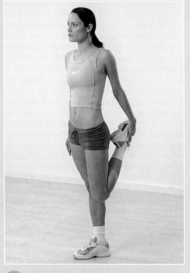 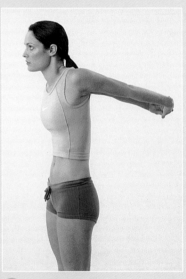

❶ calf stretch

A simple stretch for your lower leg muscles. Repeat on other side.

- Stand with hands on hips
- Take a step back
- Straighten back leg
- Face both feet forwards
- Bend front knee slightly
- Push down on your back heel
- Hold longer for a deeper stretch

❷ standing quad stretch

Keep your torso still and straight for this. Repeat on other side.

- Stand upright on one leg
- Clasp other foot behind back
- Pull foot towards buttocks
- Draw knee in and down
- Keep hips facing forwards
- Push hips forwards for a deeper stretch

❸ chest stretch

The chest area stores unwanted tension, which can cause postural problems. Use this stretch to release the tension.

- Stand upright with feet hip-width apart
- Clasp hands behind back (don't tilt forwards)
- Straighten arms
- Raise hands up

workout to a high level that will give you the benefits that you want from exercising, but your heart, lungs, and muscles have to work very hard to achieve this effort. It is because of this factor that you need to make sure that you take the time to slowly bring your body back down to a state of rest. Now the cool-down can play the same role of damage limitation in the post-exercise period.

During exercise, the constant contracting action of the muscles makes them tighter and shorter. Without stretching, the danger is that the muscles can become overly tight and remain shortened, which can then create problems within the muscle, or across the skeleton due to an imbalance in the muscles on opposing sides of the body. This can be easily prevented by making sure that you work

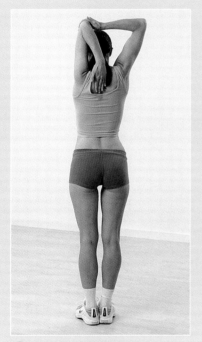 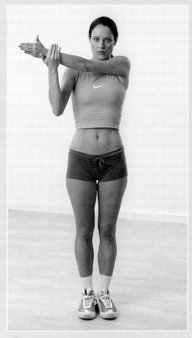 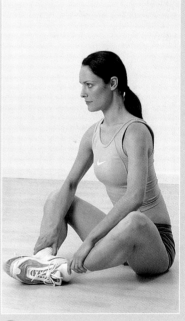

4 tricep stretch

Feel this stretch down the back of your arm. Repeat on other side.

- Stand with feet hip-width apart
- Raise left arm up
- Bend the elbow
- Position left hand behind back
- Press elbow back with right hand

5 shoulder stretch

One more isolated stretch for the shoulders to maintain flexibility. Repeat on other side.

- Stand with feet hip-width apart
- Bring straight left arm across body at chest height
- Press right hand against left arm for deeper stretch

6 adductor stretch

An effective stretch for the inner thighs. Keep your back straight.

- Sit on the floor
- Place soles of feet together
- Hold ankles
- Pull feet towards you
- Relax knees down
- Ease torso forwards from hips
- Hold longer for a deeper stretch

all parts of the body evenly during the workout, and then stretching all the muscle groups thoroughly afterwards.

Lactic acid, which is produced by the body during periods of strenuous exercise, can also build up in the muscles. Stretching the main muscles after a workout can help to disperse this lactic acid and prevent muscle spasms and injury.

Stretching effectively

The cool-down routine illustrated here contains all the essential stretches that you need to perform every time you complete one of the PHA workouts in the book. Do these stretches while your muscles are still warmed up and therefore more responsive. Each stretch should be held for a minimum of 15 seconds. Whilst holding the stretch, you should

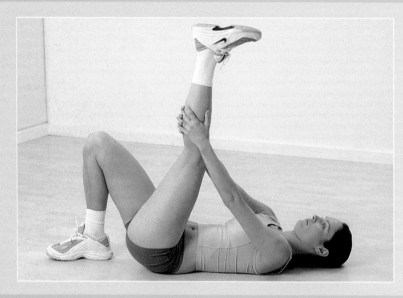

7 prone hamstring stretch

The straighter you keep your leg, the more effective this stretch will be for your hamstrings.

- Lie on your back on the floor
- Raise left leg in the air
- Hold the back of your calf
- Pull your leg gently towards you
- Hold longer for a deeper stretch, then swap legs

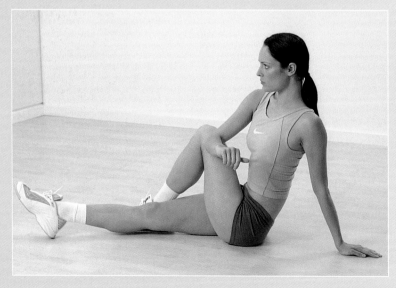

9 abductor stretch

Feel this stretch in your outer thigh muscles.

- Sit upright on the floor with legs straight
- Lift left foot over the right leg
- Keep your left knee bent
- Press the back of your left thigh with your right elbow
- Hold longer for a deeper stretch, then swap legs

actually experience the muscle relaxing, and you may even feel as if it is getting longer. If you have more time to stretch, focus on those muscles that are worth giving a little more attention to: the hamstring, calf, and adductor muscles. These are all muscles that most commonly tighten up during a normal day's activity, and, when tight, can have a real effect on your posture. With these muscle groups, you should hold the initial 15-second stretch, then aim to take the stretch a little further to intensify the effects. Hold this deeper stretch for another 15 seconds before increasing the stretch a little more and then releasing it.

Stretching can be very relaxing, so experiment with more stretches if you wish, and take longer to stretch and relax if you have the time.

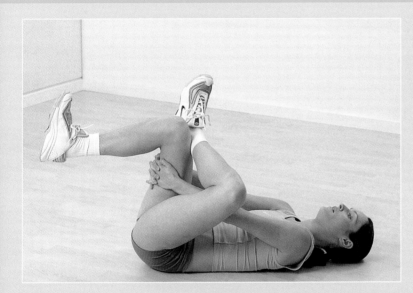

8 prone glute stretch

An essential stretch for the largest of the leg muscles.

- Lie on your back on the floor
- Bend your knees
- Rest left foot against your right knee
- Hold the back of your right thigh
- Gently pull your right leg towards you
- Hold longer for a deeper stretch, then swap legs

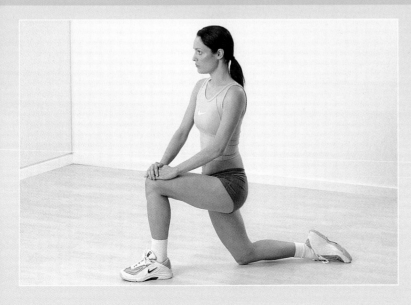

10 hip flexor

This kneeling lunge will help to prevent stiffness in the hip area.

- Kneel upright on the floor
- Step forwards with left foot
- Straighten your back
- Place your hands on your knee
- Push your hips forwards
- Hold, then swap legs

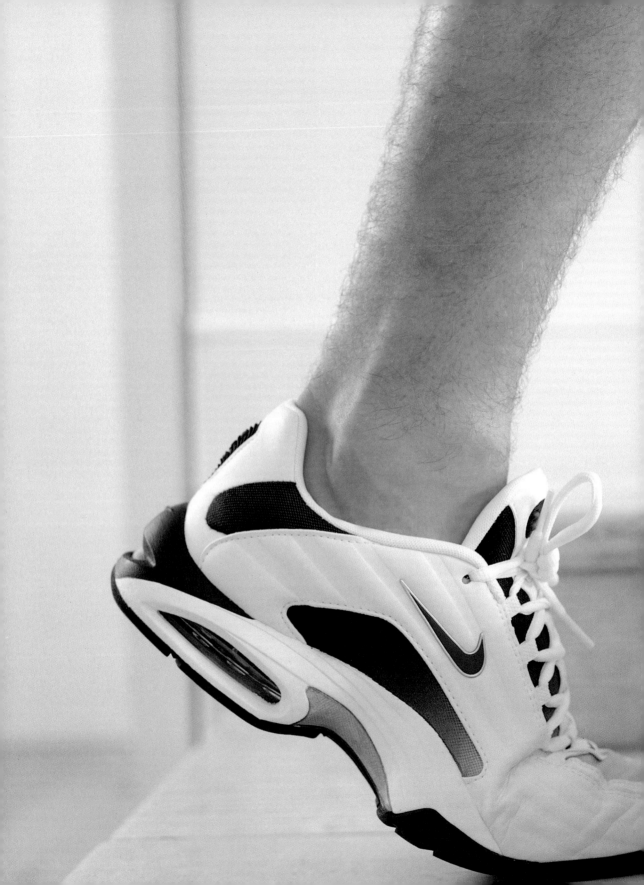

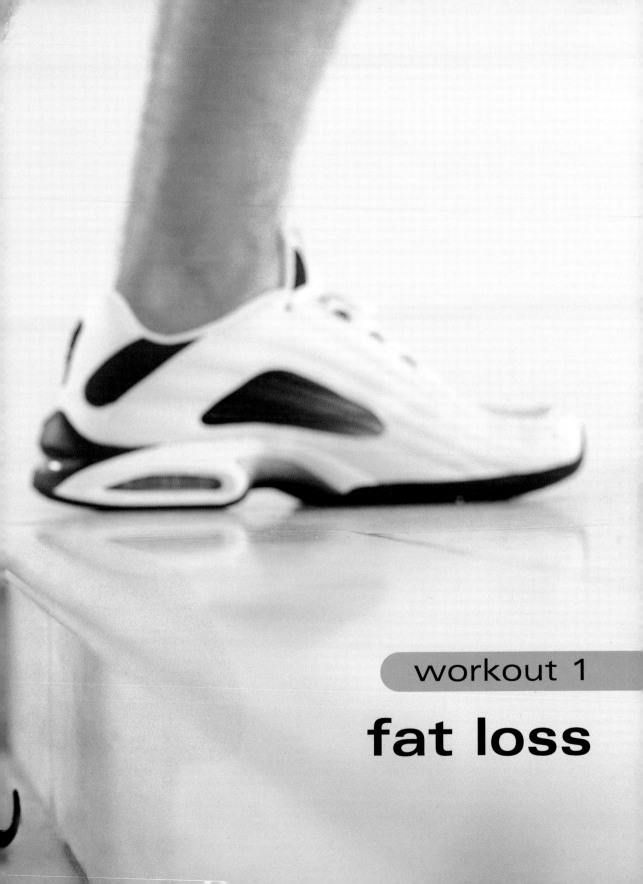

workout 1

fat loss

fat loss programme

The primary goals of the PHA Fat loss programme are to get your heart working at a higher rate in order to burn calories, and to increase the "activity" of your muscle fibres so that every muscle group is toned and conditioned.

PHA training fulfils these goals beautifully: the result of your heart working hard to supply blood to muscles at either end of your body is that you'll raise your metabolic rate (p.10) to keep burning more calories for longer, and you'll have a fit body.

How the programme works
The kind of workout that I have created for the Fat loss programme requires you to use an enormous number of muscle groups in a short

power lunges, step-ups, side leg lifts, and step-jogs. While they don't strictly follow the pattern of alternating between the upper and lower body on every single exercise, they create the same impact because your rest time in between each exercise is extremely short. Therefore, they still produce the same effects as a pure PHA programme.

You'll also be using two muscle areas – one from the lower body and one from the upper body – twice within each "mini-circuit" of repeated exercises. When this sequence is combined with the dynamic exercises, you will really feel as though you are working aerobically. If you follow the programme exactly, your heart rate will be within its ideal training zone of 75–80%MHR and you'll be burning fat effectively.

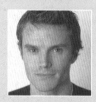

Consistency is king in the Fat loss workout if you want great results

Targeting your muscle groups
The exercises in this workout are organized so that the programme gradually works its way round from the front of the body to the

space of time, and the variety of repetitions that I have given for each exercise ensures that you will be stimulating the various muscle fibres that exist within each muscle group. Put simply, every muscle fibre you have will be made to burn calories for you, rather than sitting dormant.

When you look at how the programme is structured (right), you will notice that in between doing your PHA routine of alternating upper and lower body, I have thrown in some highly dynamic and intensive aerobic exercises, which are designed to ensure that you have a continuously high working heart rate throughout the programme. These dynamic exercises are

sides, and then to the back, ensuring that every muscle group is utilized. What we want to avoid is too much muscle fatigue, which may impair your ability to keep on the move throughout the duration of this workout. The number of repetitions you perform, and the constant variety of exercises in the flow of the programme, should stop too much fatigue occurring in any one area. So the way this programme is designed will ensure that you stay totally on the mark the entire time.

Consistency is king in the Fat loss programme: if you keep moving through this programme at the same rate for 20 minutes, you'll achieve a high-quality performance that will reap great results.

workout 1 – four times a week for six weeks

warm-up (*pp.16–19*)

exercise	level 1 reps/time	level 2 reps/time	level 3 reps/time
box press-up	20	25	30
seated squat	20	25	30
step-up	1 minute each leg	1 minute each leg	1 minute each leg
box press-up	20	25	30
seated squat	20	25	30
power lunge	30 secs each leg	30 secs each leg	30 secs each leg
lateral raise	15 rm	18 rm	20 rm
leg raise	20 secs each leg	25 secs each leg	30 secs each leg
side-leg lift	30 secs each leg	30 secs each leg	30 secs each leg
lateral raise	15 rm	18 rm	20 rm
leg raise	20 secs each leg	25 secs each leg	30 secs each leg
step-jog	30 secs each leg	45 secs each leg	1 minute each leg
reverse flye	15 rm	15 rm	15 rm
ball squat	20 reps	25 reps	30 reps
step-up	1 minute each leg	1 minute each leg	1 minute each leg
reverse flye	15 rm	15 rm	15 rm
ball squat	20 reps	25 reps	30 reps
power lunge	30 secs each leg	30 secs each leg	30 secs each leg
shoulder press	20 rm	20 rm	20 rm
ball hamstring curl	20 reps	25 reps	30 reps
side-leg lift	30 secs each leg	30 secs each leg	30 secs each leg
shoulder press	20 rm	20 rm	20 rm
ball hamstring curl	20 reps	25 reps	30 reps
step-jog	30 secs each leg	45 secs each leg	1 minute each leg
basic crunch	30 reps	40 reps	50 reps
reverse curl	20 reps	25 reps	30 reps

cool-down (*pp.20–23*)

The weights on this plan are self-adjusting: gradually increase your weights by about 10 per cent as you gain in strength. Do not exceed the number of reps listed. For alternative Fat loss travel workout, see pages 46–47.

repetition (rep): a complete exercise, from start to finish. **repetition maximum (rm):** a specific number of reps for weight-related exercises, in which the muscles become so fatigued that the last few reps are hard to perform.

fat loss visual overview

For alternative travel exercises, see pages 46–47

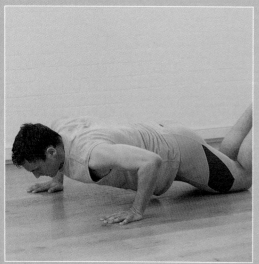

1 box press-up *p.30*

20 reps | 25 reps | 30 reps

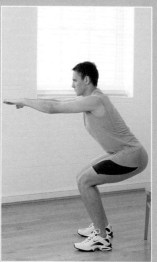

2 seated squat *p.31*

20 reps | 25 reps | 30 reps

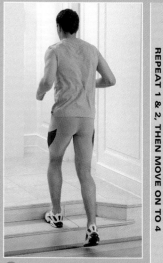

3 step-up *p.32*
(each leg)

1 min | 1 min | 1 min

REPEAT 1 & 2, THEN MOVE ON TO 4

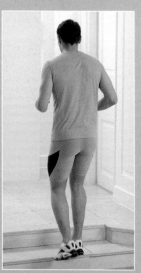

8 step-jog *p.37*
(each leg)

30 secs | 45 secs | 1 min

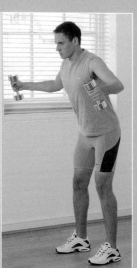

9 reverse flye *p.38*

15 rm | 15 rm | 15 rm

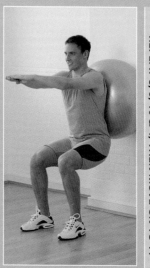

10 ball squat *p.39*

20 reps | 25 reps | 30 reps

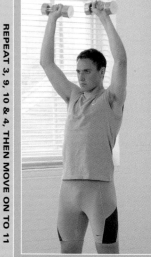

11 shoulder press *p.40*

20 rm | 20 rm | 20 rm

REPEAT 3, 9, 10 & 4, THEN MOVE ON TO 11

key | level 1 | level 2 | level 3

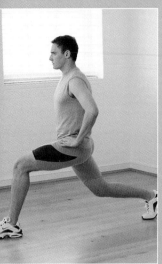

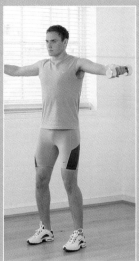

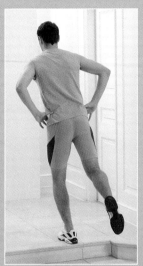

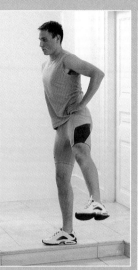

REPEAT 5 & 6, THEN MOVE ON TO 8

④ **power lunge** *p.33* (each leg)

30 secs	30 secs	30 secs

⑤ **lateral raise** *p.34*

15 rm	18 rm	20 rm

⑥ **leg raise** *p.35* (each leg)

20 secs	25 secs	30 secs

⑦ **side-leg lift** *p.36* (each leg)

30 secs	30 secs	30 secs

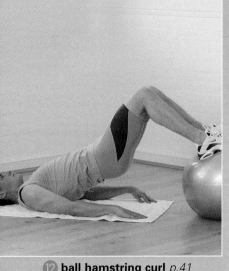

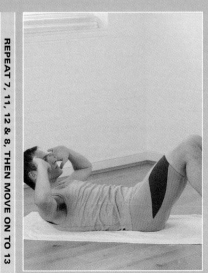

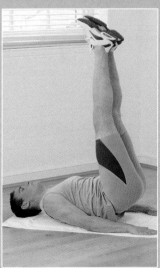

REPEAT 7, 11, 12 & 8, THEN MOVE ON TO 13

⑫ **ball hamstring curl** *p.41*

20 reps	25 reps	30 reps

⑬ **basic crunch** *p.42*

30 reps	40 reps	50 reps

⑭ **reverse curl** *p.43*

20 reps	25 reps	30 reps

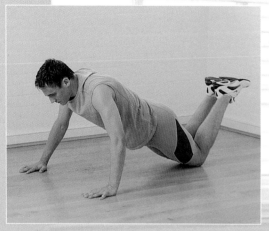

① box press-up

An adapted version of a full press-up (*p.97*), this first exercise will give you a head start toning your pecs. Make sure that your fingers face forwards, your body weight is over your hands, your back is flat, and that your abs are tight. Keep up a good pace as you work.

level 1	20 reps
level 2	25 reps
level 3	30 reps

▲ step 1

- Kneel on all fours on the floor
- Position hands just wider than shoulder-width apart
- Keep knees together on floor and raise feet in air

▼ step 2

- Inhale and lower torso down to floor until elbows are at 90°
- Exhale and push back up to start position

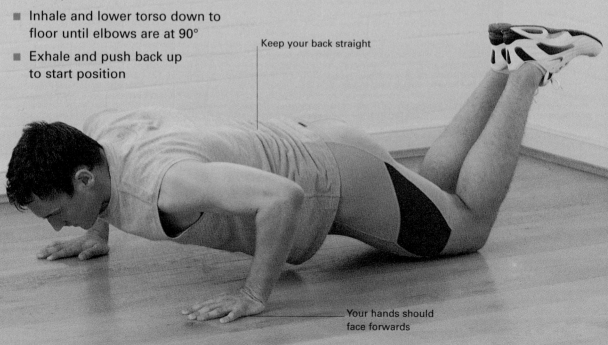

Keep your back straight

Your hands should face forwards

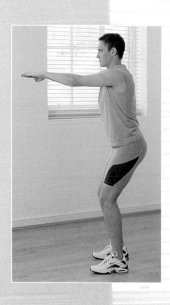

step 1

- Stand with feet hip-width apart in front of a chair
- Bend knees slightly
- Extend arms out in front of you
- Look ahead

② seated squat

This is a great lower body exercise as it tones your thighs, buttocks, and lower leg muscles all at once, giving you lean, firm legs. Use a chair – not too low – to gauge how low to squat.

level 1	20 reps
level 2	25 reps
level 3	30 reps

step 2

- Inhale and bend knees until your bottom touches the chair
- Your knees should be bent at 90°
- Keep heels on the floor
- Exhale and return to start position

31

3 step-up

Keep up the pace and do these step-ups as quickly and as energetically as you can. Change your leading foot after one minute.

level 1	1 minute each leg
level 2	1 minute each leg
level 3	1 minute each leg

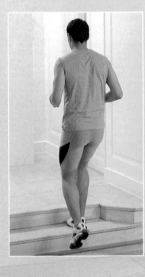

◄ step 1

- Stand facing steps
- Straighten your back
- Step up onto first step with right foot
- Place your whole foot flat on the step

► step 2

- Step up with left foot
- Place your whole foot flat on the step
- Step down, right foot first, then left foot
- Breathe evenly throughout
- Once your fitness has improved, start stepping up two steps at a time instead of one

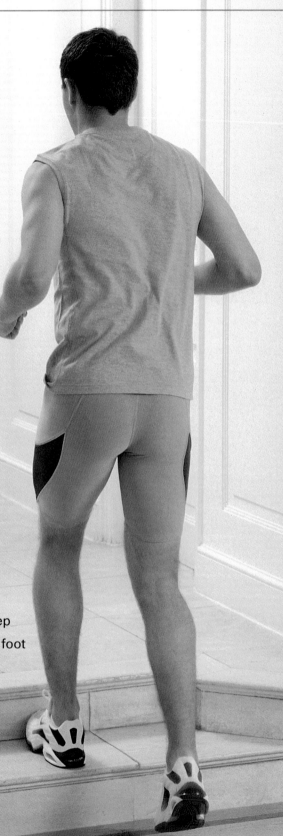

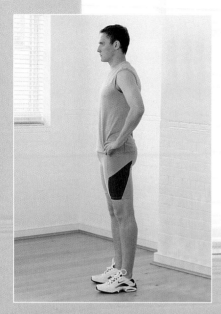

4 power lunge

To tone your inner thighs and buttocks effectively, take two or three seconds to lower down, and the same on the way up. Hold dumbbells if you want to increase the challenge. Complete 30 seconds on one leg before swapping sides.

level 1	30 secs each leg
level 2	30 secs each leg
level 3	30 secs each leg

▲ step 1

- Stand upright with feet hip-width apart
- Put hands on hips
- Look straight ahead, not down
- Take a stride forwards with one foot

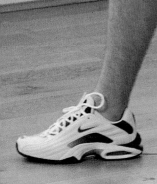

▲ step 2

- Inhale and lower back knee down towards floor
- Bring front knee directly over front foot
- Exhale and push back up to start position

Your weight should be on the heel of your front foot

Keep your palms facing down and don't let your hands twist round

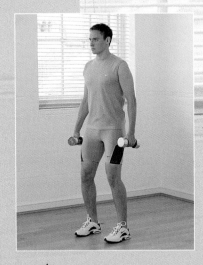

⑤ lateral raise

For this exercise, you'll switch once again to working your upper body. Use dumbbells to provide you with enough resistance to create well-toned shoulder muscles.

level 1	15 rm
level 2	18 rm
level 3	20 rm

▲ step 1

- Hold dumbbells with palms facing your sides
- Position feet hip-width apart
- Bend knees slightly
- Straighten your back
- Tighten abs

◄ step 2

- Exhale and slowly raise arms out to the sides
- Keep elbows slightly bent
- Keep torso still
- Stop when hands reach shoulder level
- Inhale and slowly lower arms down to start position

⑥ leg raise

This exercise may look simple, but it really tests your quads and hamstrings. Use the second step of a flight of stairs or steps to make each leg raise dynamic. Start with the left leg first, then the right leg.

level 1	20 secs each leg
level 2	25 secs each leg
level 3	30 secs each leg

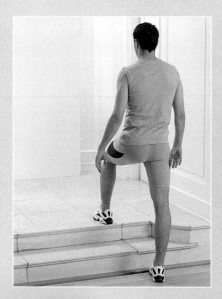

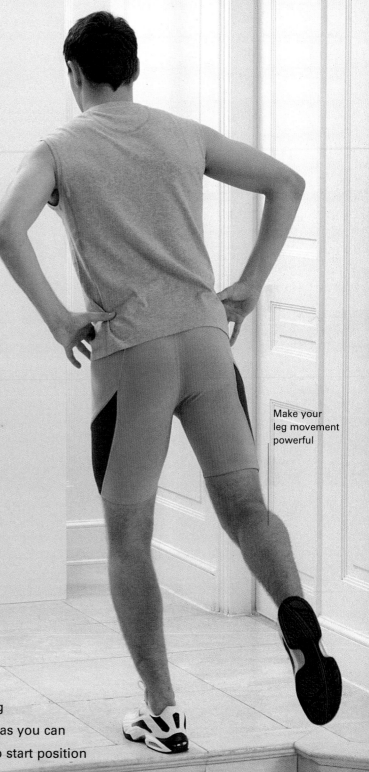

Make your leg movement powerful

▲ step 1

- Place left foot on second step
- Straighten back and tighten abs

▶ step 2

- Step up and put weight onto left leg
- Raise right leg behind you, as high as you can
- Hold for two seconds, then lower to start position

7 side leg-lift

This movement uses your body weight as resistance to tone the legs. Complete 30 seconds on one leg, then swap sides.

level 1	30 secs each leg
level 2	30 secs each leg
level 3	30 secs each leg

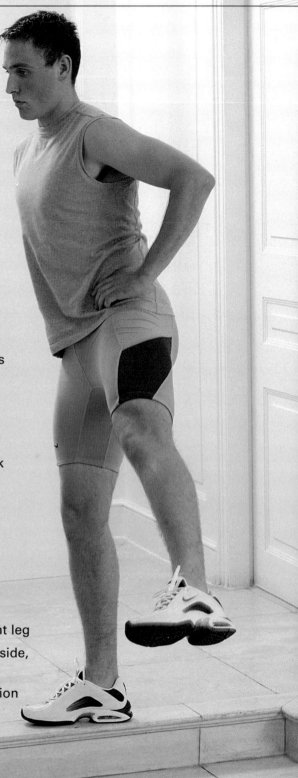

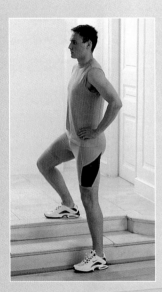

◄ step 1

- Stand at right angles to steps
- Place right foot on second step
- Place hands on hips
- Straighten your back
- Tighten abs

► step 2

- Put weight onto right leg
- Raise left leg out to side, as high as you can
- Return to start position
- Breathe evenly throughout

(8) step-jog

Up the ante with this fast-paced exercise: it will not only work your lower body, it'll raise your heart rate to keep burning the calories. Change your leading foot halfway through.

level 1	30 secs each leg
level 2	45 secs each leg
level 3	1 minute each leg

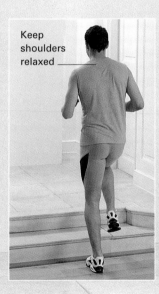

Keep shoulders relaxed

◄ ## step 1

- Stand in front of some steps
- Straighten your back
- Step up with right foot
- Place your whole foot flat on the step

► ## step 2

- Step up with left foot
- Both feet should be flat on the step
- Step down, right foot first, then left foot
- Repeat immediately without pause, one second up, one second down
- Breathe evenly throughout

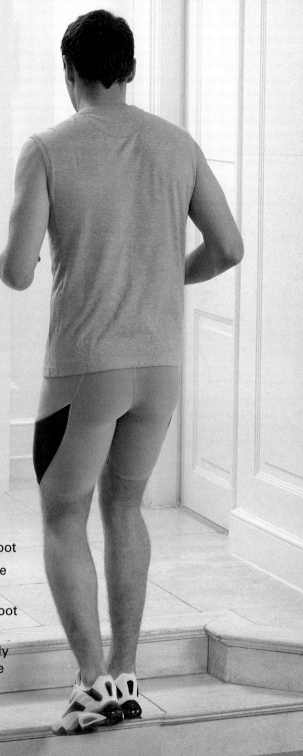

Relax your shoulders; don't let them hunch forwards

9 reverse flye

This demanding exercise yields great results for an under-used area of the body. The reverse flye targets your posterior deltoids, leaving you looking toned and feeling strong. Avoid curving your back upwards as you lift the weights.

level 1	15 rm
level 2	15 rm
level 3	15 rm

▲ step 1

- Stand with feet hip-width apart and knees bent
- Straighten your back and lean forwards from hips
- Hold dumbbells and extend arms down in front of you

◄ step 2

- Exhale and raise arms up and out to each side
- Maintain body posture
- Keep arms almost straight
- Squeeze shoulder blades together
- Inhale and slowly lower arms down to start position

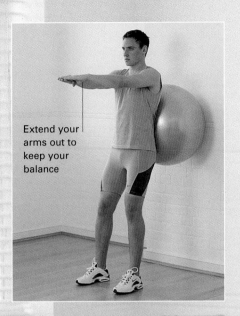

Extend your arms out to keep your balance

10 ball squat

Back to a lower body exercise to strengthen and shape your legs, and still burn the calories. Control your movements to get the maximum impact.

level 1	20 reps
level 2	25 reps
level 3	30 reps

▲ step 1

- Stand in front of a wall
- Position fitness ball between lower and middle back
- Lean against wall
- Your legs should be almost fully extended, with your feet slightly ahead of your body
- Keep back straight

▶ step 2

- Inhale and slowly lower torso down
- Stop when thighs are at 90°
- Hold position briefly
- Exhale and push up to start position

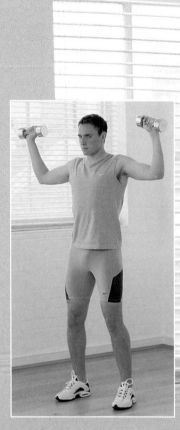

⑪ shoulder press

Keep the momentum going and move quickly onto this upper body exercise. Standing up to perform the shoulder press increases the workload on your abs and postural muscles. You can, if you want to, perform the exercise sitting down, with your back well supported, to concentrate the workload onto your deltoids.

level 1	20 rm
level 2	20 rm
level 3	20 rm

▲ step 1

- Hold a dumbbell in each hand
- Stand with feet hip-width apart
- Bend knees slightly
- Extend arms out to sides at shoulder level
- Bend elbows 90°
- Tighten abs

◀ step 2

- Exhale and press dumbbells upwards until arms are almost straight
- Keep torso still
- Inhale and lower down to start position
- Count one second up, one second down

⑫ ball hamstring curl

This exercise looks simple, but it's great for toning the backs of the thighs. Keep your hips raised throughout the exercise to make the action even more intense, and press your hands down on the floor to stabilize yourself.

level 1	20 reps
level 2	25 reps
level 3	30 reps

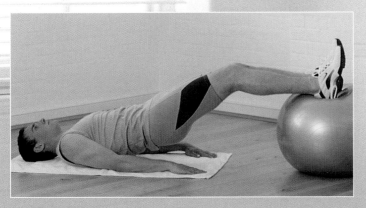

◁ step 1

- Lie on your back on a mat
- Press heels into middle of ball
- Extend legs, position feet together, and point toes
- Keep your arms by your sides, palms face down
- Lift hips off ground

▽ step 2

- Exhale and tighten abs
- Pull ball slowly towards you until your feet are flat on the ball
- Keep head, shoulders, and back on floor
- Inhale and push ball back to start position

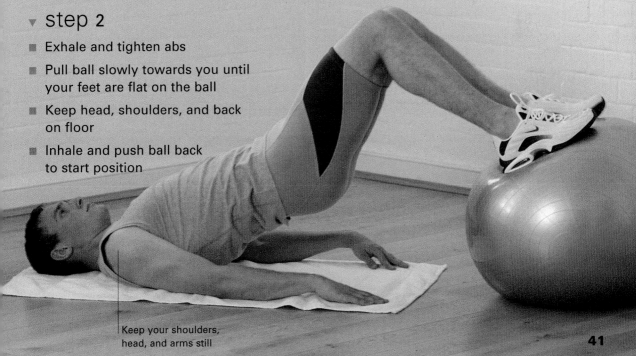

Keep your shoulders, head, and arms still

41

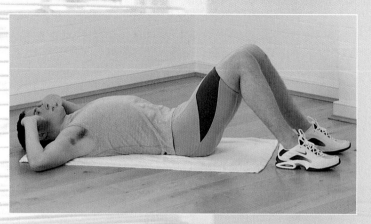

⑬ basic crunch

This standard exercise is great for toning and defining the stomach muscles. Keep your moves slow and controlled.

level 1	30 reps
level 2	40 reps
level 3	50 reps

▲ step 1

- Lie on back, knees bent, feet flat on floor
- Place hands at the sides of your head
- Inhale and really tighten abs

▼ step 2

- Exhale and raise shoulders off floor
- Keep a gap between chin and chest
- Hold for one second, keeping your neck relaxed
- Inhale and lower back down to start position

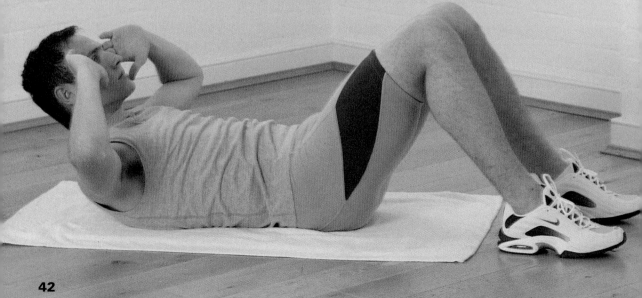

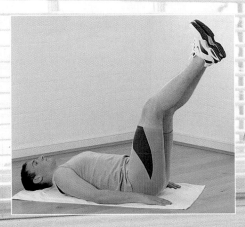

⑭ reverse curl

This may feel like a bit of a killer to end the workout, but stick with it and you'll soon have fantastically toned abs.

level 1	20 reps
level 2	25 reps
level 3	30 reps

▲ step 1

- Lie on your back on a mat
- Press palms onto floor
- Raise legs in the air

▼ step 2

- Tighten lower abs and exhale
- Curl legs and pelvis towards chest
- Keep legs at 90° to torso
- Keep head and shoulders on floor
- Inhale and slowly return to start position

Your legs should be straight

Keep your back flat on the floor at all times

43

questions & answers

Beginning any fitness programme inevitably raises questions that you may not have thought about before, and issues that you feel you need answers to. Here are my responses to a few of the most common questions that my clients ask me about their health, losing weight, and getting fit.

Q **What can I do if I want to fit in more exercise than the Fat loss programme prescribes?**

a All the fitness programmes in this book are designed to be as complete as you'll need for you to achieve your own personal goals. If you have the time and you want to do some more exercise, then there is no harm in adding in extra cardiovascular exercise to your routine. You can run or row, for example, for 30–40 minutes three or four times a week in addition to performing a PHA workout. However, I do not suggest adding any more weights-based exercises to your weekly PHA programme, since you may end up not giving your muscles enough recovery time in between sessions for them to be able to adapt and increase in strength (p.152).

Q **I'm exercising every other day now, but I also want to eat more too. Is this normal?**

a Any increase in your activity levels will result in your body needing more fuel. However, your body may tend to over-compensate for this, and want more than it actually needs. This can result in unwanted weight gain. I have witnessed people in training for a marathon actually gaining weight, simply because they thought that the training they were doing

gave them free rein to eat whatever they wanted, whenever they wanted. On the days that you train, you'll probably notice that a couple of hours after you've finished your workout you'll develop an insatiable appetite. The key to avoiding these hunger pangs is to make sure that you eat some protein and carbohydrate during the 30-minute post-training period, such as a deep-filled chicken or tuna sandwich, or some oatcakes with cottage cheese or houmous (*for other snack options, see p.153*). Eating at this time will aid your recovery from training and help you to avoid any feelings of ravenous hunger later on in the day.

Q **I'm doing the Fat loss workout, and eating healthily, but I don't seem to have much energy at the end of the week. Why is this?**

a Starting a new, healthier diet and an exercise routine at the same time can often lead to an initial feeling of fatigue. Persevere, though, and you will soon start to feel more energized. Your body is adapting to the different types of "fuel" that you are eating, as well as the new physical demands you are making on it. Combine these elements with a busy lifestyle, and it's no wonder that your energy is flagging by the end of the week. What you must make sure of is that you're not attempting to do too much. Stick to the suggested Fat loss exercise

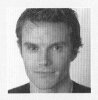

Don't be discouraged if you haven't lost weight for a week; keep trying and you'll get there

programme, don't exceed it (more isn't always better), and make sure that you are honest with yourself about your real level of fitness when you start exercising: if you have any doubts about how fit you really are, begin at the lowest level. Finally, make sure that you are drinking enough water during the day, as this can have a dramatic effect on your energy levels.

Q Will a high-protein diet assist me in doing any of the exercise programmes in this book?

a No, high-protein diets, such as the Atkins diet, will not help you to get the best out of these PHA workouts. Such diets are not to be recommended if you are interested in living a healthy lifestyle, since they deplete the body of essential nutrients and won't supply you with enough energy to perform any exercise programme. High-protein diets are not healthy, and they are certainly not the answer to achieving longevity and a greater sense of well-being. A balanced approach to your eating habits is, quite simply, the best kind of diet available.

Q I've lost a little weight initially, but now I have done the workout for four weeks I just can't seem to lose any more weight. Should I repeat the Fat loss programme all over again?

a If this is the case, you should repeat the programme again, and this time, make sure that you are working your muscles intensively and applying the correct techniques. You've also got to ensure that your heart rate is remaining at a high rate throughout the workout, so invest in a heart rate monitor (*p.158*), or keep checking your pulse (*p.19*). People often find that weight loss happens in phases as their body adjusts, or if their body's fluid retention or fluid loss varies on a week-by-week basis. Don't be discouraged if you haven't lost weight for a week or so: the weight will shift again. Keep on trying hard with every workout and you'll keep getting closer to your goal.

Q I've lost some weight, but not much has changed around my thighs and my waistline. Should I double the reps for some exercises?

a Don't change the programme at all, as it is designed to enable you to achieve your goals in the most productive way possible. If you are carrying excess fat around the waistline, for instance, it is likely that this is your "sticky" area, which means that you'll see results in that particular part of your body last. It is not because the exercises aren't working, it is just that you have a greater number of fat cells in that area, which need to be reduced. And this will happen, all in good time.

45

fat loss travel alternative

The beauty of the PHA Fat loss programme is that it can be performed at home with just a couple of dumbbells and a fitness ball. However, though the exercises "travel" well if you go away, the equipment is not sufficiently light or small enough to pack into a suitcase. By replacing this equipment with an exertube (*p.158*) and substituting a few exercises, you'll be able to work out wherever you go.

1 box press-up, p.30

2 seated squat, p.31

3 step-up, p.32

4 power lunge, p.33

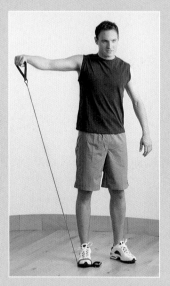

5 **single-arm lateral raise**

- Stand with feet hip-width apart
- Wrap end of exertube around right foot
- Grasp handle in right hand, palm facing inwards, and tighten abs
- Exhale and slowly lift right arm out to shoulder height
- Inhale and lower down to start position
- Levels 1/2/3 = 10/15/20 reps each side

6 leg raise, p.35

7 side-leg lift, p.36

8 step-jog, p.37

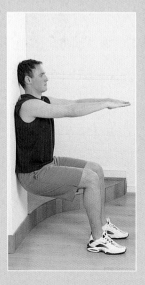

10 **wall sit**

- Lean against a wall
- Position feet a short distance from the wall
- Inhale and lower torso down until thighs are at 90° to floor
- Hold for 20–40 seconds, depending on fitness
- Inhale and push up

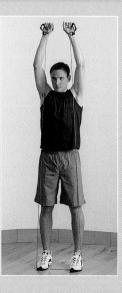

11 **shoulder press**

- Stand on exertube, feet hip-width apart
- Grasp handles, bend elbows 90° and position hands at shoulder height
- Exhale and raise arms up above head
- Avoid locking arms straight
- Inhale and lower down to start position
- Levels 1/2/3 = 15/20/25 reps

| key | ① see main workout |
| | ① travel alternative |

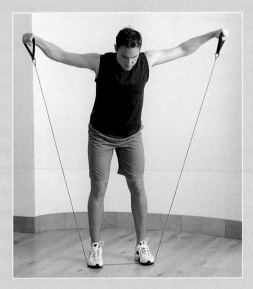

⑨ reverse flye

- Stand on exertube, feet hip-width apart
- Grasp handles with palms facing towards you
- Lean forwards slightly with back straight
- Exhale and raise arms out and away from sides
- Lift handles up to shoulder height, keeping arms almost straight
- Inhale and lower down to start position
- Levels 1/2/3 = 10/15/20 reps

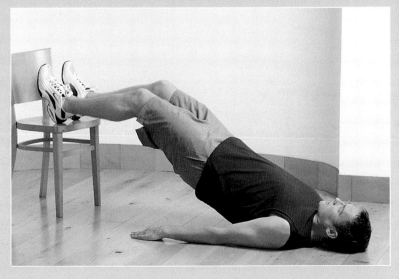

⑫ body lift

- Lie on back on the floor, arms at sides
- Rest feet on chair
- Exhale and raise pelvis until torso is in a straight line
- Inhale and lower down to start position
- Levels 1/2/3 = 20/25/30 reps

⑬ basic crunch, p.42

⑭ reverse curl, p.43

fat loss training log

Writing down everything that you achieve in your workouts can be really motivating, especially if you begin to see real improvements. Photocopy these pages and keep a log of every workout you do.

exercise	date: weight	reps	date: weight	reps	date: weight	reps
box press-up set 1						
seated squat set 1						
step-up set 1						
box press-up set 2						
seated squat set 2						
power lunge set 1						
lateral raise set 1						
leg raise set 1						
side-leg lift set 1						
lateral raise set 2						
leg raise set 2						
step-jog set 1						
reverse flye set 1						

Keep moving, and you'll be **burning fat** effectively

exercise (continued)	weight	reps	weight	reps	weight	reps
ball squat set 1						
step-up set 2						
reverse flye set 2						
ball squat set 2						
power lunge set 2						
shoulder press set 1						
ball hamstring curl set 1						
side-leg lift set 2						
shoulder press set 2						
ball hamstring curl set 2						
step-jog set 2						
basic crunch set 1						
reverse curl set 1						

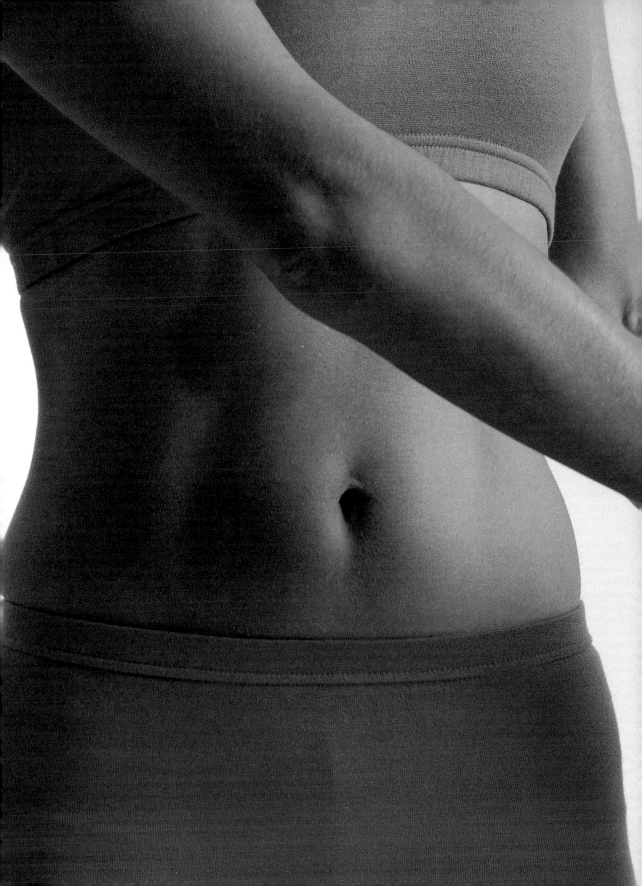

muscle-sculpting

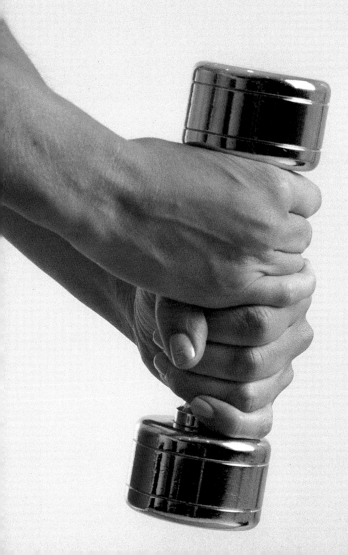

muscle-sculpting programme

Achieving good muscle tone is not just about looking and feeling stronger, it's about reducing body fat, looking leaner and taller, and improving posture. I've designed this workout to challenge your entire body and to make you feel that you look better, whether clothed or naked! By applying the PHA technique to the selected resistance exercises, you'll achieve a sculpted look in half the usual time.

The PHA challenge

Not only will we be using the PHA system of alternating between the upper and lower body muscles for every exercise on this programme,

Pumping your muscles

By grouping the exercises in this programme into sets of four, with each set performed twice in quick succession before a brief rest, you'll be working your muscles to the point where they become "pumped" and so retain their firmness for some time. Working around and then down the body will make you feel that each area of your body is being pushed to its limit, but not quite beyond. Thus the workout feels achievable, yet also very testing. One of the benefits of PHA training is continuing fat reduction as a result of the calories you'll burn, so you'll also look slimmer and fitter.

 This a **total body workout, where you'll be testing** every **muscle**

we'll also be alternating between muscle groups at the front and the back of the body. This extreme fluctuation of blood demand between all areas of the body in a short period of time is the key to ensuring that you challenge as many muscle groups as possible in short, isolated "hits".

If you are worried about gaining muscle bulk rather than muscle tone, rest assured: on this workout you won't be overloading any one area of your body enough to run the risk of building any muscle size, and you won't be using very heavy weights. However, I can guarantee that you'll be working your muscles to an optimum level so that they'll become firmer and leave you looking leaner.

Keeping a balance

This is a total body workout, so don't be surprised if you feel fatigued at the end of a session. You'll be testing every fibre in every main muscle of the body. The mistake that people often make in trying to sculpt their body is that they focus too much on individual areas, which then doesn't provide them with a well-balanced body, or they use weights that are too heavy in the expectation that they can produce significant results in a shorter time frame. Using heavy weights could well make you bulky – unless you know how to use them sparingly, and in the correct way. Concentrating on what you perceive to be your worst body areas can often lead you to create shape, and sometimes too much size, in small areas of the body, while other areas are overlooked. Stick to this plan, however, and you'll soon have a great body that you can be proud of.

workout 2 – four times a week for six weeks

warm-up (*pp.16–19*)

exercise	level 1 reps	level 2 reps	level 3 reps
chest press	20 rm	20 rm	20 rm
power lunge	15 each leg	20 each leg	25 each leg
lateral pull-down	20 rm	20 rm	20 rm
hamstring curl	20 rm	20 rm	20 rm

repeat set above, then rest for 30 secs before beginning next set below

pec flye	20 rm	20 rm	20 rm
seated squat	20	25	30
seated row	20 rm	20 rm	20 rm
ball hamstring curl	15	20	30

repeat set above, then rest for 30 secs before beginning next set below

single-arm pull-down	20 rm each arm	20 rm each arm	20 rm each arm
glute raise	20 each leg	25 each leg	30 each leg
tricep dip	15	20	25
advanced crunch	25	30	40

repeat set above, then rest for 30 secs before beginning next set below

bicep curl	20 rm	20 rm	20 rm
static bridge leg lift	10 each leg	15 each leg	20 each leg
tricep push-down	15 rm	15 rm	15 rm
reverse curl	20	25	30

repeat set above, then rest for 30 secs before beginning next set below

single-arm lateral raise	15 rm each arm	15 rm each arm	15 rm each arm
jump squat	15	20	25
back extension	15	20	30
body lift	20	25	30

repeat set above, then rest for 30 secs

cool-down (*pp.20–23*)

The weights on this plan are self-adjusting: gradually increase your weights by about 10 per cent as you gain in strength. Do not exceed the number of reps listed. For an alternative Muscle-sculpting travel workout, see pages 78–81.

repetitions (reps): the complete performance of an exercise from start position to finish position.
repetition maximum (rm): a specific number of reps for weight-related exercises, in which the muscles become so fatigued that the last few reps are hard to perform.

muscle-sculpting visual overview

For alternative travel exercises, see pages 78–81

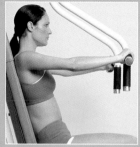

1 **chest press** *p.56*

20 rm	20 rm	20 rm

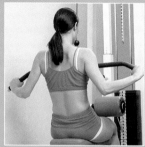

2 **power lunge** *p.57* (each leg)

15 reps	20 reps	25 reps

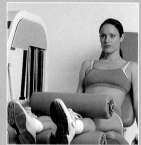

3 **lateral pull-down** *p.58*

20 rm	20 rm	20 rm

4 **hamstring curl** *p.59*

20 rm	20 rm	20 rm

REPEAT 1–4 + 30-SEC REST

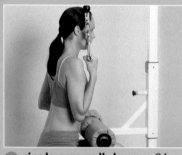

9 **single-arm pull-down** *p.64* (each arm)

20 rm	20 rm	20 rm

10 **glute raise** *p.65* (each leg)

20 reps	25 reps	30 reps

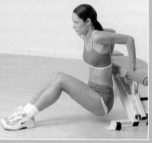

11 **tricep dip** *p.66*

15 reps	20 reps	25 reps

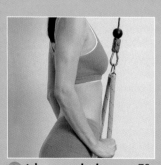

15 **tricep push-down** *p.70*

15 rm	15 rm	15 rm

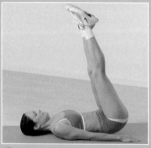

16 **reverse curl** *p.71*

20 reps	25 reps	30 reps

REPEAT 13–16 + 30-SEC REST

17 **single-arm lateral raise** *p.72* (each arm)

15 rm	15 rm	15 rm

key	level 1	level 2	level 3

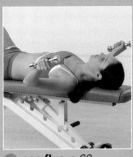 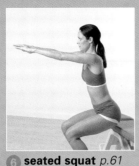 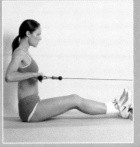 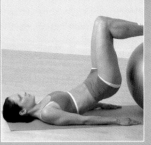

REPEAT 5–8 + 30-SEC REST

⑤ **pec flye** *p.60*　　⑥ **seated squat** *p.61*　　⑦ **seated row** *p.62*　　⑧ **ball hamstring curl** *p.63*

20 rm	20 rm	20 rm	20 reps	25 reps	30 reps	20 rm	20 rm	20 rm	15 reps	20 reps	30 reps

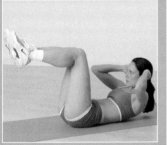 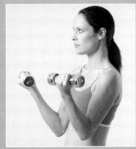 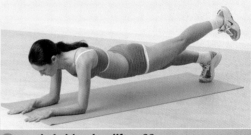

REPEAT 9–12 + 30 SEC REST

⑫ **advanced crunch** *p.67*　　⑬ **bicep curl** *p.68*　　⑭ **static bridge leg lift** *p.69* (each leg)

25 reps	30 reps	40 reps	20 rm	20 rm	20 rm	10 reps	15 reps	20 reps

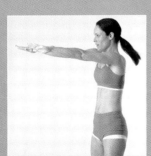 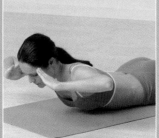 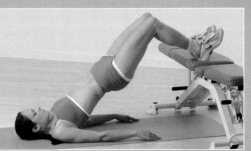

REPEAT 17–20 + 30-SEC REST

⑱ **jump squat** *p.73*　　⑲ **back extension** *p.74*　　⑳ **body lift** *p.75*

15 reps	20 reps	25 reps	15 reps	20 reps	30 reps	20 reps	25 reps	30 reps

1 chest press

The chest press machine builds strength and shape in your chest area and triceps. Keep your movements controlled and powerful.

level 1	20 rm
level 2	20 rm
level 3	20 rm

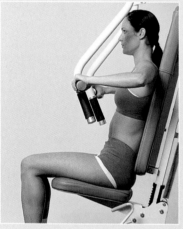

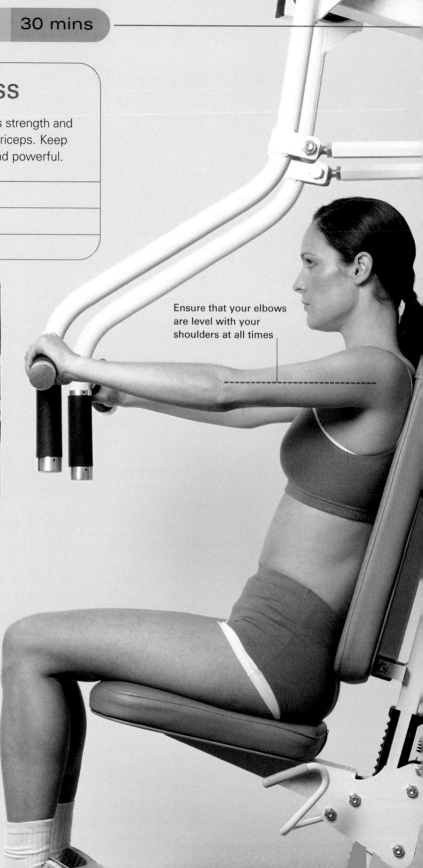

Ensure that your elbows are level with your shoulders at all times

▲ step 1

- Sit at chest press machine with lower back supported
- Grasp the handles
- Bend elbows to 90°

▶ step 2

- Exhale and push forwards until arms are almost fully extended
- Inhale and return arms to start position
- Count four seconds for each repetition

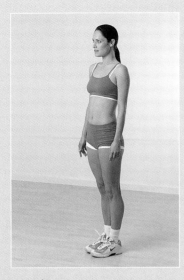

2 power lunge

This effective exercise tones your inner thighs and buttocks; use dumbbells if you want to make it even more of a challenge. Don't let your front knee travel beyond your toes as you lunge down. Alternate your legs with each rep.

level 1	15 reps each leg
level 2	20 reps each leg
level 3	25 reps each leg

▲ step 1

- Stand upright
- Relax arms at sides or place hands on hips
- Tighten abs
- Look straight ahead

◄ step 2

- Inhale and take a stride forwards
- Lower back knee down towards the floor
- Position front knee directly above front foot
- Exhale and push back up to start position

Keep body weight over heel of front foot

③ lateral pull-down

Move quickly on to this upper body exercise, which works the large muscles of the back. Keep your back straight and strong as you pull against the resistance of the weights.

level 1	20 rm
level 2	20 rm
level 3	20 rm

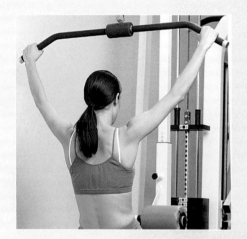

▲ step 1

- Sit at lat pull-down machine
- Hold bar firmly with hands wider than shoulder-width apart
- Straighten your back and tighten abs

Don't lean back as you pull down

▶ step 2

- Exhale and pull down for two seconds
- Inhale and return to start position, taking a total of four seconds per repetition

(4) hamstring curl

Switch back to a lower body exercise to keep your heart rate up. This machine works the hamstring muscles. Keep your lower back well supported throughout.

level 1	20 rm
level 2	20 rm
level 3	20 rm

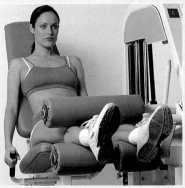

▲ step 1

- Sit at leg curl machine with legs extended
- Rest ankles on roller pads
- Position large roller pad over shins

▶ step 2

- Exhale and bend legs for two seconds
- Push your heels towards your buttocks
- Inhale and return to start position for two seconds

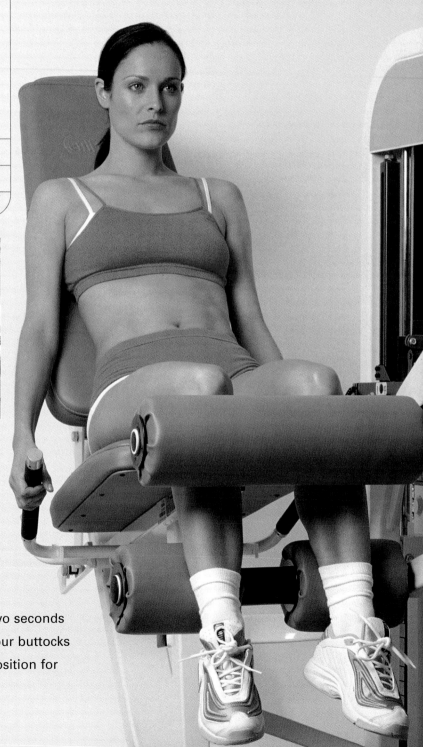

⑤ pec flye

This next upper body exercise strengthens and defines the pectoral chest muscles. Good technique is essential, so check regularly that your moves are accurate.

level 1	20 rm
level 2	20 rm
level 3	20 rm

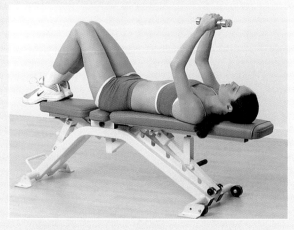

▲ step 1

- Lie back on an exercise bench
- Position feet at the end of the bench, or flat on the floor
- Hold a dumbbell in each hand
- Extend arms up above chest

When your arms are extended, your elbows should be at 90° to your sides

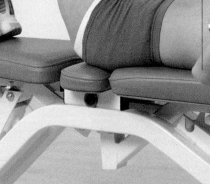

▲ step 2

- Inhale and lower arms out to sides until almost fully extended
- Squeeze pecs and exhale
- Slowly return to start position

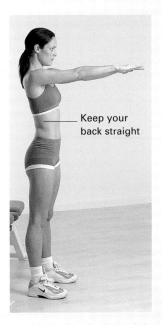

Keep your
back straight

6 seated squat

Use an exercise bench as a marker so that you bend your knees properly. Your bottom should touch the edge of the bench as you squat.

level 1	20 reps
level 2	25 reps
level 3	30 reps

▲ step 1

- Stand in front of an exercise bench

- Position feet hip-width apart

- Extend arms out in front of you

- Straighten your back

◄ step 2

- Inhale and bend knees until thighs are parallel with floor

- Keep looking ahead

- Exhale and push back up to standing position

Keep your heels on
the floor throughout

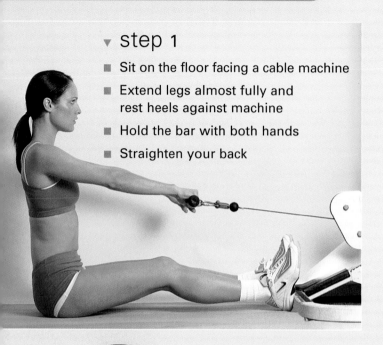

▼ step 1

- Sit on the floor facing a cable machine
- Extend legs almost fully and rest heels against machine
- Hold the bar with both hands
- Straighten your back

⑦ seated row

Using a cable machine for this exercise will enable you to sculpt the muscles of your upper and middle back. To get the maximum benefit, keep your torso and legs as still as possible while you power away with your arms.

level 1	20 rm
level 2	20 rm
level 3	20 rm

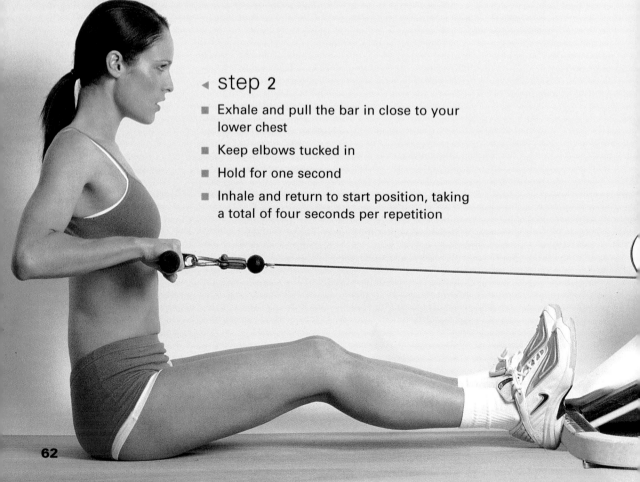

◄ step 2

- Exhale and pull the bar in close to your lower chest
- Keep elbows tucked in
- Hold for one second
- Inhale and return to start position, taking a total of four seconds per repetition

⑧ ball hamstring curl

Back to one more lower body exercise before the end of the set. Press your palms onto the floor and tighten your abs to keep your torso still, and steady the fitness ball with your feet.

level 1	15 reps
level 2	20 reps
level 3	30 reps

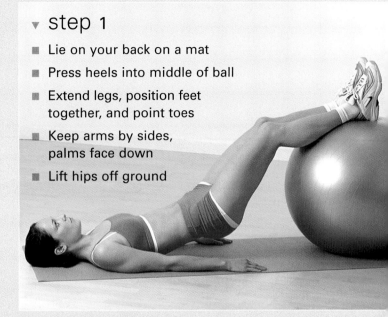

▼ step 1

- Lie on your back on a mat
- Press heels into middle of ball
- Extend legs, position feet together, and point toes
- Keep arms by sides, palms face down
- Lift hips off ground

▼ step 2

- Tighten abs and exhale
- Pull ball slowly towards you until your feet are flat on the ball
- Keep head, shoulders, and back on floor
- Inhale and push ball back to start position

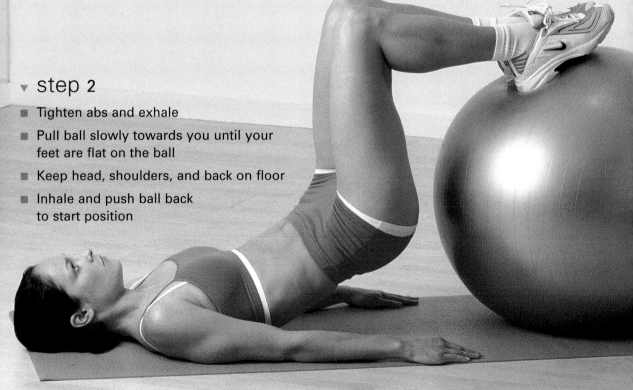

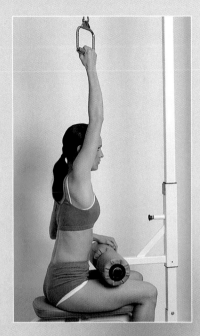

9 single-arm pull-down

Keep up the pace and target your upper back and triceps with this single-arm pull-down. Use a lat pull-down machine with a handle attachment, and adjust the weight down for this single-arm exercise. Repeat on the right, then the left, arm.

level 1	20 rm each arm
level 2	20 rm each arm
level 3	20 rm each arm

▲ step 1

- Sit at a lat pull-down machine
- Hold handle in one hand
- Extend arm almost fully above head

▶ step 2

- Keep body still
- Exhale and pull handle straight down
- Keep elbow at the side rather than in front of the body
- Bend arm until hand is level with shoulder
- Inhale and return to start position

⑩ glute raise

This exercise may look simple, but it really tests your quads and hamstrings. Control your movements to make each leg lift strong and as powerful. Complete the reps on one leg, then swap sides.

level 1	20 reps each leg
level 2	25 reps each leg
level 3	30 reps each leg

▼ step 1

- Position yourself on all fours on a mat
- Place hands shoulder-width apart
- Extend one leg out straight behind you
- Straighten your back

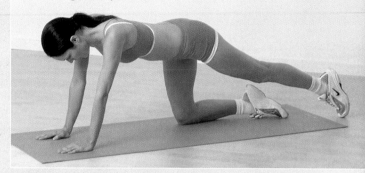

▼ step 2

- Exhale and raise extended leg up, heel first
- Keep head and neck in line with back
- Hold for one second
- Inhale and slowly lower leg

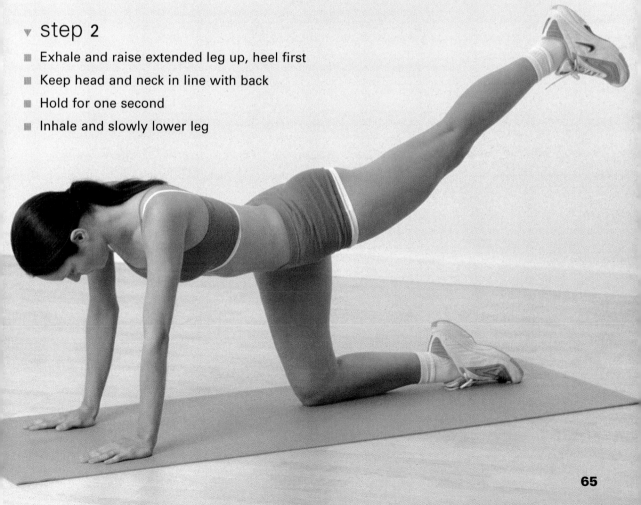

⑪ tricep dip

Transfer back to the exercise bench to work your upper arms and give your major muscle groups a brief rest. Again, good technique is essential if you want to get the best results.

level 1	15 reps
level 2	20 reps
level 3	25 reps

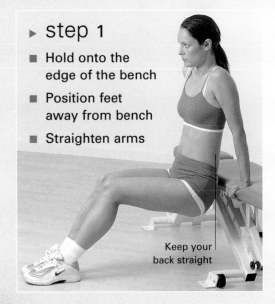

▶ **step 1**

- Hold onto the edge of the bench
- Position feet away from bench
- Straighten arms

Keep your back straight

▶ **step 2**

- Inhale and lower torso down until your elbows are at 90°
- Exhale and slowly push yourself back up
- Don't lock your arms at the top of the movement

Keep your body close to the bench

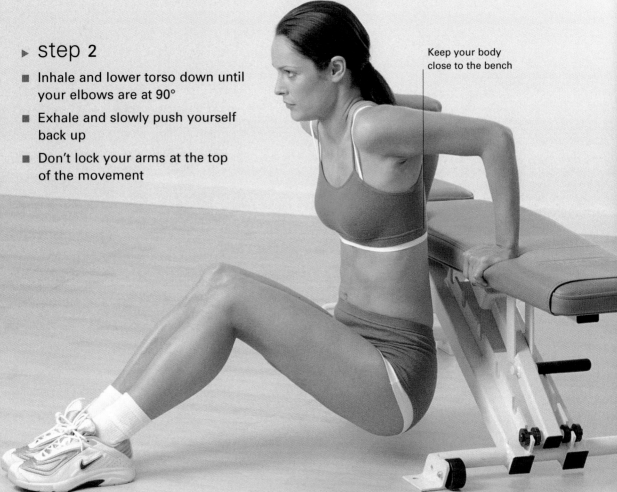

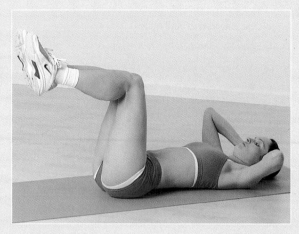

⑫ advanced crunch

This version of the crunch works all the muscles in the abdominal area, so stick with it and you'll see fantastic results. Keep your knees bent and feet off the floor throughout.

level 1	25 reps
level 2	30 reps
level 3	40 reps

▲ step 1

- Lie on your back on a mat
- Raise feet off the floor
- Bend knees 90°
- Place your fingers at the sides of your head
- Tighten abs and exhale

▼ step 2

- Lift shoulder blades off the floor
- Curl shoulders forwards
- Press lower back onto floor
- Inhale and lower down to start position

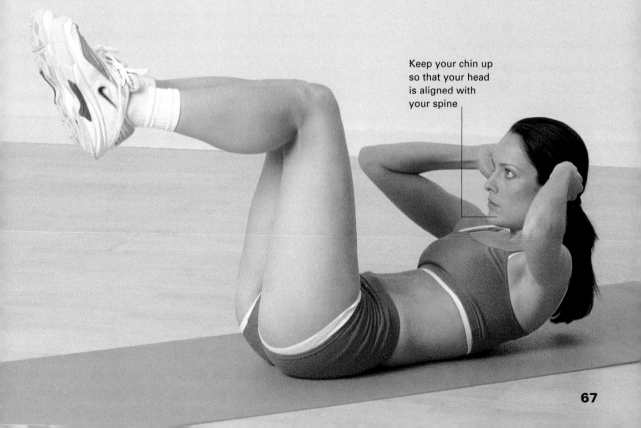

Keep your chin up so that your head is aligned with your spine

⓭ bicep curl

This intensive exercise for your upper arms gives them great definition and strength. Flexing your biceps while holding the dumbbells will help to "pump" and firm the muscles.

level 1	20 rm
level 2	20 rm
level 3	20 rm

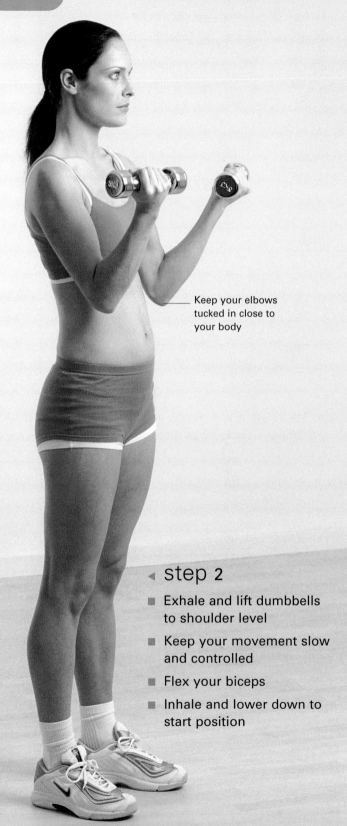

Keep your elbows tucked in close to your body

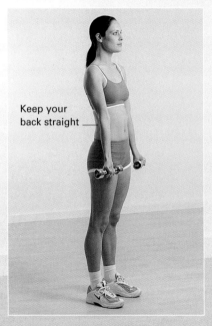

Keep your back straight

▲ step 1

- Hold a dumbbell in each hand
- Stand with feet hip-width apart
- Bend knees slightly
- Face your palms forwards

◄ step 2

- Exhale and lift dumbbells to shoulder level
- Keep your movement slow and controlled
- Flex your biceps
- Inhale and lower down to start position

⑭ static bridge leg lift

This is a tough balancing exercise that targets your waistline, but it produces great results. If you wobble as you raise your leg, check that you have tight abs. Start with a small lift until you get your balance, then build up to a 30 cm (12 in) leg lift. Alternate your leg lifts to give each leg a very brief rest.

level 1	10 reps each leg
level 2	15 reps each leg
level 3	20 reps each leg

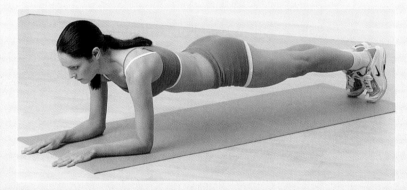

◄ step 1

- Lie on your front on a mat
- Position elbows under shoulders
- Balance on your elbows, forearms, and toes
- Straighten your back

▼ step 2

- Tighten abs, exhale, and raise one leg up
- Keep your back straight
- Inhale and lower down to start position

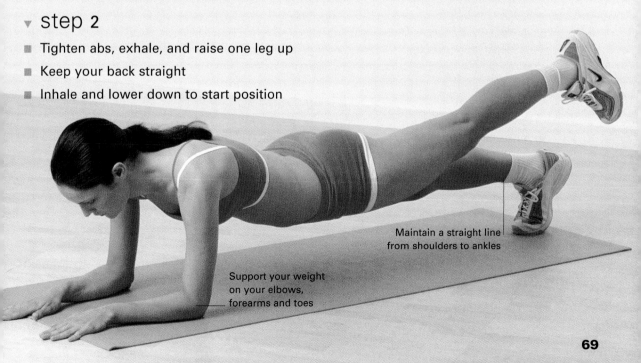

Maintain a straight line from shoulders to ankles

Support your weight on your elbows, forearms and toes

⑮ tricep push-down

Back to another upper body exercise to keep your heart rate up. This exercise targets the backs of your arms. Squeeze your triceps as you pull down on the rope handle attachment to create muscle definition.

level 1	15 rm
level 2	15 rm
level 3	15 rm

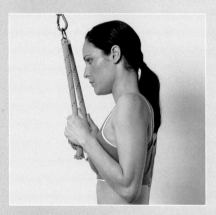

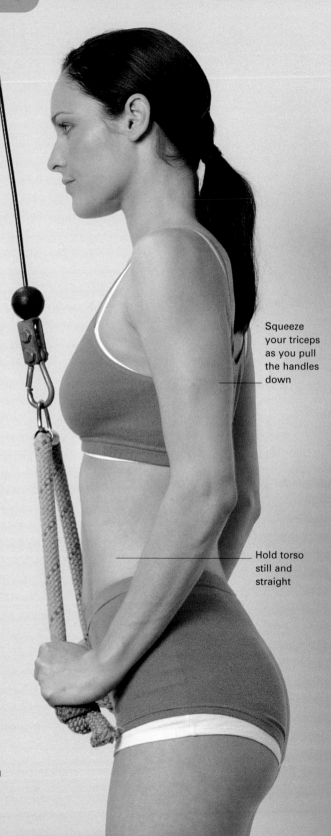

Squeeze your triceps as you pull the handles down

Hold torso still and straight

▲ step 1

- Stand in front of a cable machine with feet hip-width apart
- Grasp rope handles at shoulder height and keep elbows tucked in

▶ step 2

- Exhale and push handles down until arms are almost fully extended
- Move hands outwards as you pull
- Inhale and release up to start position

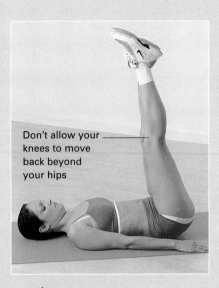

Don't allow your knees to move back beyond your hips

⑯ reverse curl

Use the strength of your lower abs rather than the momentum of your legs here, and control your moves so that you don't throw your legs over your body.

level 1	20 reps
level 2	25 reps
level 3	30 reps

▲ step 1

- Lie on your back on a mat
- Press palms onto floor
- Raise legs straight in the air

▶ step 2

- Tighten lower abs and exhale
- Curl legs and pelvis towards chest
- Keep legs at 90° to torso
- Keep head and shoulders on floor
- Inhale and slowly release down to start position

Keep your
torso still

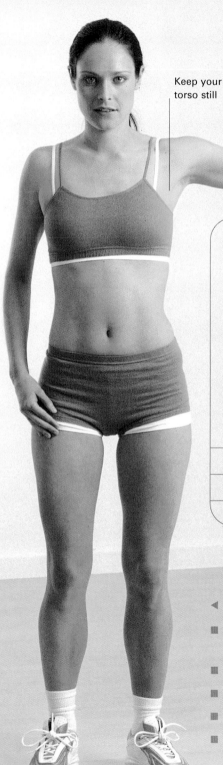

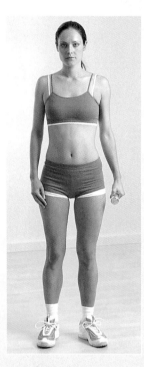

⑰ single-arm lateral raise

This exercise is worth doing in front of a mirror to check that your technique is correct. The action of raising the dumbbell utilizes all three sections of your deltoids to sculpt your shoulder area effectively. Do all the reps on one arm, then change sides and repeat.

level 1	15 rm each arm
level 2	15 rm each arm
level 3	15 rm each arm

▲ **step 1**

- Hold dumbbell in left hand, palm facing inwards
- Stand with feet hip-width apart
- Bend knees slightly
- Relax right arm at your side

◄ **step 2**

- Exhale and slowly raise arm out to side
- Keep elbow slightly bent
- Raise dumbbell to shoulder level
- Keep palm facing down
- Inhale and slowly lower to start position

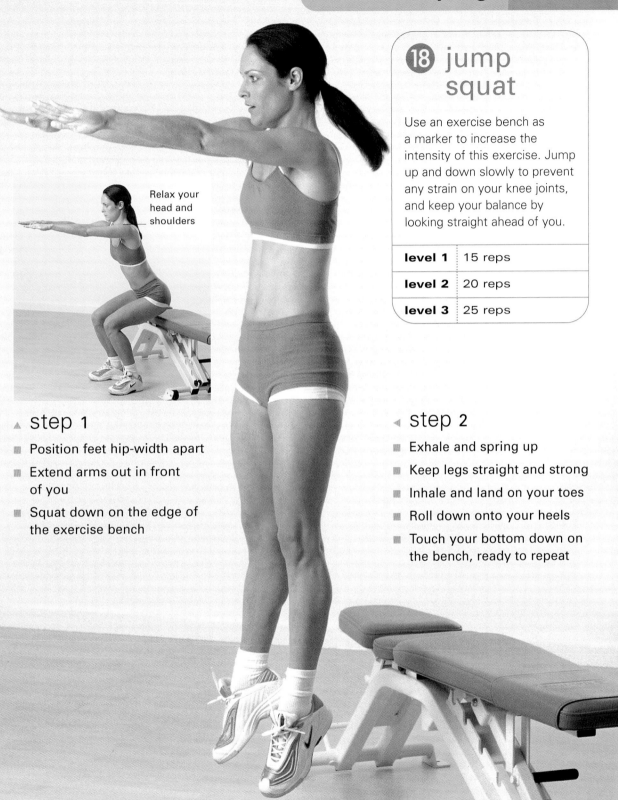

⑱ jump squat

Use an exercise bench as a marker to increase the intensity of this exercise. Jump up and down slowly to prevent any strain on your knee joints, and keep your balance by looking straight ahead of you.

level 1	15 reps
level 2	20 reps
level 3	25 reps

Relax your head and shoulders

▲ step 1

- ▦ Position feet hip-width apart
- ▦ Extend arms out in front of you
- ▦ Squat down on the edge of the exercise bench

◀ step 2

- ▦ Exhale and spring up
- ▦ Keep legs straight and strong
- ▦ Inhale and land on your toes
- ▦ Roll down onto your heels
- ▦ Touch your bottom down on the bench, ready to repeat

73

▼ step 1

- Lie on your front on a mat
- Place your hands at the sides of your head
- Point toes

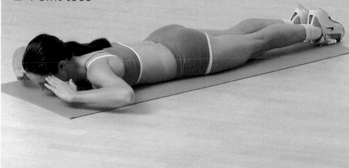

⑲ back extension

A strong back is vital if you are lifting weights, so build up the strength in your back with this exercise. It's also a fantastic way of improving your posture. Maintain slow, controlled movements at all times to get the maximum benefit.

level 1	15 reps
level 2	20 reps
level 3	30 reps

▼ step 2

- Exhale and raise head and upper body off floor
- Keep hips and toes pressed onto floor
- Hold for one second
- Inhale and lower down to start position

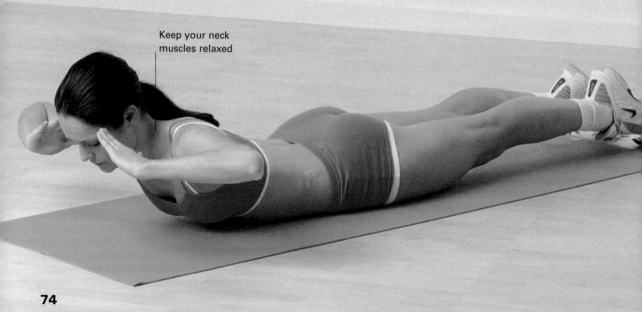

Keep your neck muscles relaxed

▼ step 1

- Lie on your back on a mat
- Rest heels on the edge of an exercise bench
- Place palms face down on the floor

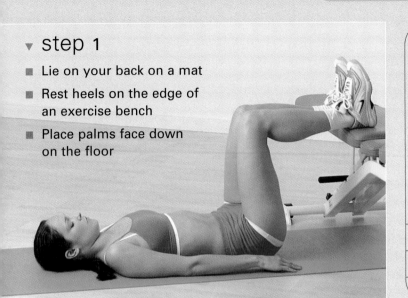

⑳ body lift

This final exercise is an intensive workout for your buttocks and the backs of your legs. Make the muscles work even harder by pointing your toes away from you. Grit your teeth and power your way through this last one.

level 1	20 reps
level 2	25 reps
level 3	30 reps

▼ step 2

- Exhale and raise pelvis right up
- Squeeze buttocks hard
- Inhale and slowly lower down to start position

Your body should be straight from your knees to your chest _____

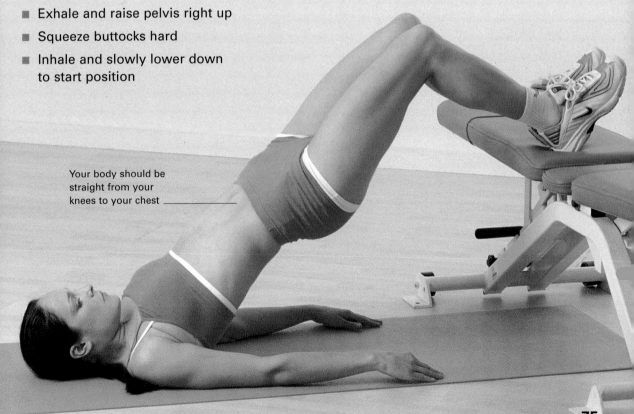

questions & answers

The words "muscle-sculpting" may make you feel as though you'll have to be prepared to change your body image completely, and perhaps become someone you're not. If you feel daunted about doing resistance training with weights, don't worry, the answers below should help to reassure you.

Q   I'm worried that I might gain too much muscle on the Muscle-sculpting programme. Will this happen to me?

a One of the most common fears that people, and women especially, have about resistance training is that as soon as they start lifting weights, they will gain more muscle than they wish for and end up looking bulky. This fear is completely understandable, but gaining large muscles is actually very difficult to do, and particularly so for women, since they have lower testosterone levels than men.

The basic rule to help you achieve a toned look and avoid building large muscles is to follow an exercise programme that uses light weights and high repetitions – as outlined in the Muscle-sculpting programme. This workout will enable you to create lean, defined muscles rather than thick, bulky muscles, and then stay that way.

One other factor to be aware of when you embark on a programme of resistance exercise such as this is that, before you start to lose body fat, you may begin to see some muscle definition. Areas of body fat lie over muscle tissue, so it may feel as though your body is getting bigger to begin with. However, you'll soon start getting the toned, athletic look you're aiming for if you stick with the workout and do it four times a week. Concentrate on burning calories to lessen your body fat, and with patience and faith your toned look will appear.

Q   How should my muscles feel when I'm working out on this resistance programme?

a You should aim to work your muscles hard while you are following the Muscle-sculpting programme. With each set of exercises, you should feel as though your muscles are being pushed to their limit and reaching the point of overload (*below*). For example, if you are performing a bicep curl for 20 repetitions, the last three to four reps should feel difficult to complete. If you feel like you could keep going for longer, check that your technique is correct.

Q   What exactly is muscle overload, and can it damage your muscles?

a Muscle overload refers to the process of pushing the body beyond its normal physical limitations. The point at which a muscle reaches the limits of its capability is when it "fails" to be able to complete a set of repetitions, and then becomes increasingly less effective during successive sets. This signals that the muscle is overloaded. The process of overloading causes "positive muscle trauma", in which the body is pushed to adapt and become fitter to cope with the extra effort required. Overload sounds extreme, but it is a crucial part

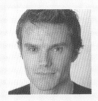

The **Muscle-sculpting plan** will enable you to create **lean, defined muscles**, not thick, bulky muscles

of everybody's fitness development. You should aim to achieve overload whenever you work out if you want to get great results.

Q **If I want to train for longer than the Muscle-sculpting programme recommends, can I do so?**

a If you are thinking of adding some aerobic work to this programme, I would advise doing no more than three to four sessions of 30–40 minutes each time. This would give you quite a considerable weekly programme, so you will need to have plenty of energy and eat enough calories to keep you going. There is certainly no harm in doing more work: the fact is that the PHA system gives you time to do more because it has already halved your normal resistance workout time.

Q **Is it worth buying any of the sports energy drinks on the market, or should I stick to drinking just water?**

a As a general rule for any training programme that lasts for less than 60 minutes, water is the best choice. So you shouldn't need to consider drinking anything but water while you are performing the four PHA programmes in this book. However, if you are

supplementing these workouts with cardiovascular exercise such as running or rowing, and you train for longer than an hour at a time, then some form of carbohydrate drink can be a good idea to keep your energy levels topped up. There are many different drinks on the market, but the key ingredient to look for in a product is a "long-chain carbohydrate", such as maltodextrin, in addition to the "shorter-chain carbohydrates", glucose and fructose. Many cheaper sports drinks contain only the latter ingredients, which, despite giving you an instant energy hit, will not provide the sustained fuel your body requires. Also, if you are exercising in the heat, it's a good idea to buy a drink containing electrolytes, as this ingredient will help to prevent dehydration more effectively than water can alone.

Q **If I become pregnant, should I stop doing my workouts immediately or can I keep exercising?**

a You'll need to seek medical advice from your doctor about your specific situation and current fitness levels. You should avoid any exercise that increases your blood pressure significantly when pregnant. For this reason, it is best to avoid the Bulking up programme when pregnant. Provided you monitor your heart rate at all times and adjust your training so that your heart doesn't rise above about 145BPM, you should be fine on the other programmes – but do take advice first.

muscle-sculpting travel alternative

I have changed some of the exercises in this travel alternative from the original muscle-sculpting programme to make it easier for you to exercise while you travel, but the outline remains the same.

Aim to perform the exercises in sets of four, doing each set twice, with a 30-second rest before starting the next set. Move swiftly between exercises to get the blood pumping quickly up and down the body.

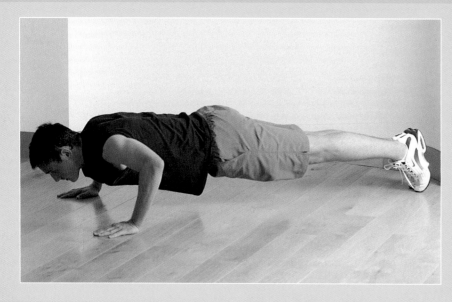

1 press-up

- Balance on toes and hands
- Position hands just wider than shoulder-width apart
- Inhale and lower torso down until elbows are at 90°
- Exhale and push up
- Levels 1/2/3 = 20/25/30 reps, or try box press-up, p.30

2 power lunge, p.57

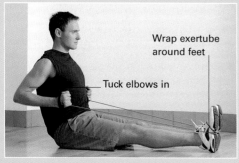

Wrap exertube around feet

Tuck elbows in

5 seated row

- Sit upright on the floor with legs straight
- Pull handles into sides of lower torso
- Levels 1/2/3 = 20/25/30 reps

6 seated squat, p.61

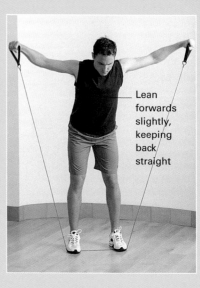

Lean forwards slightly, keeping back straight

7 reverse flye

- Stand on exertube, feet hip-width apart
- Grasp handles, palms face inwards
- Exhale and raise arms out to sides
- Lift handles up to shoulder height
- Inhale and lower to start position
- Levels 1/2/3 = 20/25/30 reps

| key | see main workout |
| | travel alternative |

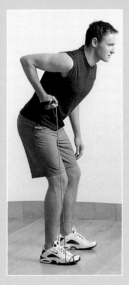

❸ single-arm row

- Wrap one end of exertube around right foot
- Grasp other handle in right hand and wrap around hand until taut
- Bend knees slightly and lean forwards a little
- Exhale and pull tube until elbow is at 90°
- Inhale and relax hand back down
- Levels 1/2/3 = 15/20/25 reps on each side

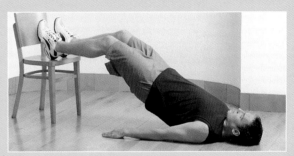

❹ body lift on chair

- Lie on back on the floor, arms at sides
- Rest feet on chair and exhale
- Raise pelvis until torso is in a straight line
- Inhale and lower down to start position
- Levels 1/2/3 = 20/25/30 reps

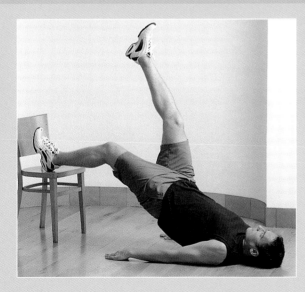

❽ single-leg body lift

- Lie on back on the floor, arms at sides
- Rest left foot on a chair
- Exhale and raise right leg in the air
- Lift pelvis until torso is in a straight line
- Inhale and lower down to start position
- Levels 1/2/3 = 15/20/25 reps each side

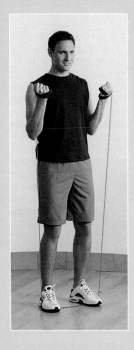

9 bicep curl

- Stand on the exertube, feet hip-width apart
- Wrap tube round hands until taut
- Face palms forwards
- Exhale and raise hands to shoulder height
- Inhale and lower hands
- Levels 1/2/3 = 15/20/25 reps

10 glute raise, p.65

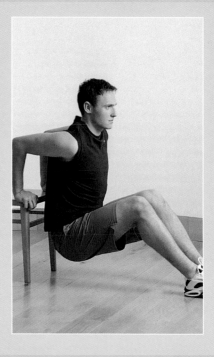

11 tricep dip

- Hold chair seat, with palms facing backwards
- Move feet away from chair
- Inhale and lower down until elbows are at 90°
- Exhale and push up until arms are almost straight
- Levels 1/2/3 = 15/20/25 reps

12 advanced crunch, p.67

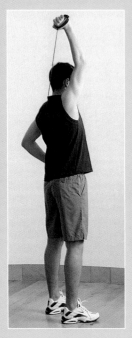

15 overhead tricep extension

- Hold centre of exertube in left hand
- Grasp handle in right hand and raise arm
- Bend elbow so that your hand is behind your back
- Exhale and extend arm
- Avoid locking your arm straight
- Inhale and lower hand
- Levels 1/2/3 = 15/20/25 reps each side

16 reverse curl, p.71

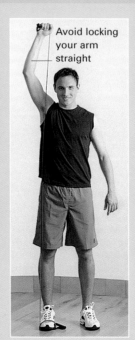

Avoid locking your arm straight

17 single-arm shoulder press

- Stand with feet hip-width apart
- Wrap end of exertube around right foot
- Grasp remaining handle in right hand and position hand at shoulder height
- Exhale and extend arm
- Inhale and return to start position
- Levels 1/2/3 = 15/20/25 reps each side

18 jump squat, p.73

19 back extension, p.74

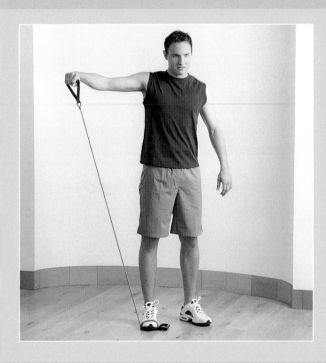

⑬ single-arm lateral raise

- Stand with feet hip-width apart
- Wrap end of exertube around right foot
- Grasp handle in right hand, palm facing inwards, tighten abs, and exhale
- Slowly lift right arm out to shoulder height
- Inhale and lower down to start position
- Levels 1/2/3 = 10/15/20 reps each side

⑭ static bridge leg lift, p.69

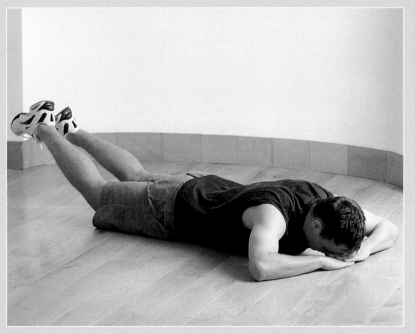

⑳ leg lift

- Lie on front on floor
- Relax shoulders and rest head on hands
- Tighten abs and exhale
- Lift both legs off the floor, as high as you can
- Inhale and relax back down
- Levels 1/2/3 = 15/20/25 reps

muscle-sculpting training log

The temptation on this programme is to keep the weights the same and increase the reps, but to see the best results you should keep increasing your weights so that the specified reps remain difficult.

exercise	date: weight	reps	date: weight	reps	date: weight	reps
chest press set 1						
power lunge set 1						
lateral pull-down set 1						
hamstring curl set 1						
chest press set 2						
power lunge set 2						
lateral pull-down set 2						
hamstring curl set 2						
pec flye set 1						
seated squat set 1						
seated row set 1						
ball hamstring curl set 1						
pec flye set 2						
seated squat set 2						
seated row set 2						
ball hamstring curl set 2						
single-arm pull-down set 1						
glute raise set 1						
tricep dip set 1						
advanced crunch set 1						

Work your **muscles hard** so that you get a **great body**

exercise (continued)	weight	reps	weight	reps	weight	reps
single-arm pull-down set 2						
glute raise set 2						
tricep dip set 2						
advanced crunch set 2						
bicep curl set 1						
static bridge leg lift set 1						
tricep push-down set 1						
reverse curl set 1						
bicep curl set 2						
static bridge leg lift set 2						
tricep push-down set 2						
reverse curl set 2						
single-arm lateral raise set 1						
jump squat set 1						
back extension set 1						
body lift set 1						
single-arm lateral raise set 2						
jump squat set 2						
back extension set 2						
body lift set 2						

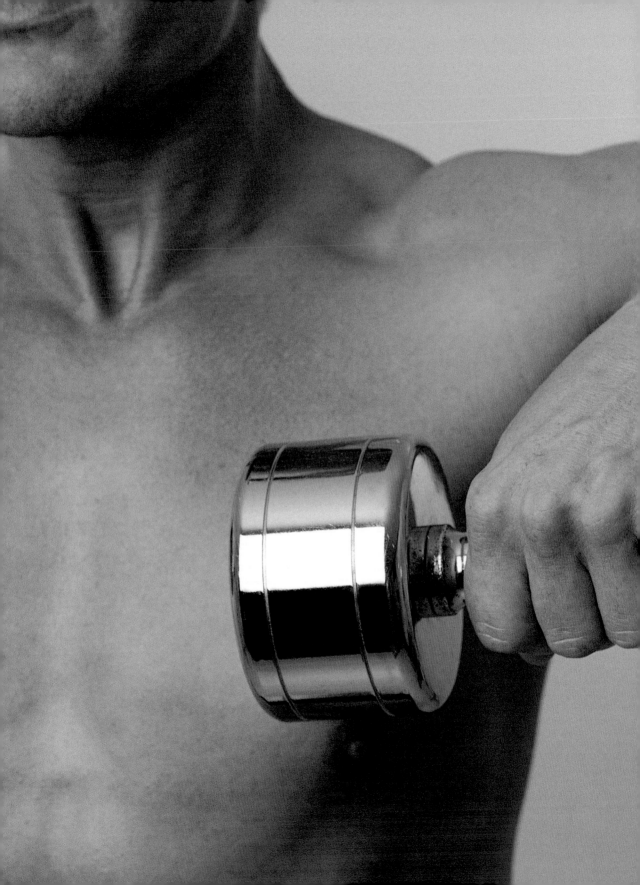

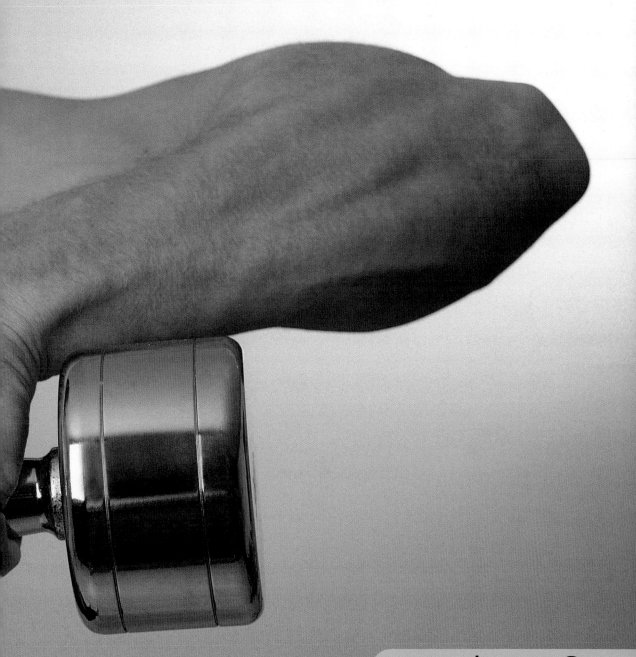

workout 3

bulking up

bulking up programme

If you want a body that's big and powerful, the hard work is about to begin – with stunning results. Building muscle is usually a time-consuming process, but on this PHA programme you'll exercise for just 40 minutes, four times a week, and still create fantastic muscle mass and definition.

Why two workouts?

By its nature, muscle-bulking works your muscles to their absolute limit, so we need to give your body a "split" routine that will allow you to rest various muscles on some days while you work other areas instead. By using two workouts twice a week in an alternating pattern, you will be able to fully overload each area individually, and then allow

large loadings of weight, we'll use an isolation exercise (when just one muscle group is used), and immediately follow it up with a compound exercise (when several muscle groups work in conjunction with one another). This back-to-back approach causes muscle fibres to be severely overloaded with a large weight during the isolation phase, and then given a second hit, with a helping hand from other muscles, in the compound exercise in order to wring every last ounce of strength from the area.

During this process, microscopic tearing occurs in the muscle fibres, which stimulates them to regenerate as stronger, more adaptable muscles, so that, as you keep training, you have a growing capacity for lifting weights.

We need to **work** every main **muscle group** of the body **intensively**

good levels of recovery for a few days before the muscles are hit again. Workout 3a works the chest, triceps, glutes, and hamstrings, while workout 3b targets the biceps, back, quads, and shoulders.

The theory behind the workouts

The approach that I have taken with this PHA programme means that you'll work a specific area of the upper body for two quick-succession, back-to-back exercises. These two exercises are rapidly followed by a single lower body exercise, which provides the PHA "blood shunt" effect that has such great benefits. As we need to work each muscle area in the upper body intensively with

Added benefits

The sheer time requirements of normal muscle-bulking routines means that people often neglect doing any cardiovascular exercise. PHA training overcomes this problem by encouraging greater cardiovascular effects than conventional resistance training does. This advantage is substantial: you have, in effect, a two-in-one workout. Dedicated muscle-bulking advocates may argue that the body needs to rest between sets, but the evidence of muscle usage on a PHA programme shows that the "active recovery" rate provided to the arms while the legs are working actually aids the dispersion of lactic acid from the muscles, which is the biggest inhibitor to additional workload on any one area.

So, on this programme you will be able to halve your muscle-bulking workout time and produce an overall body image that is highly desirable.

workout 3 – four times a week for six weeks

warm-up (*pp.16–19*)

workout 3a	reps	workout 3b	reps
pec flye	10 rm	barbell curl	10 rm
chest press	8 rm	pull-up	to failure
hamstring curl	10 rm	leg extension	12 rm
cable crossover	8 rm	hammer curl	12 rm
press-up	to failure	upright row	8 rm
dead lift	12 rm	barbell squat	10 rm
tricep extension	10 rm	seated row	10 rm
tricep dip	to failure	single-arm pull-down	10 rm each side
bench step-up	15 each leg	*repeat set above x2 then move on to set below*	
repeat set above x2 then move on to set below		lateral raise	12 rm
advanced crunch	50	power lunge	12 each leg
alternate crossover	30 each side	shoulder press	10 rm
back extension	25	fixed lunge	12 each leg
reverse leg lift	25	reverse flye	10 rm
basic crunch	50	*repeat set above x2*	
isolated crossover	30 each side		
straight-leg crunch	40		
repeat set above x2			

cool-down (*pp.20–23*)

Workouts 3a and 3b in *Bulking up* are two 40-minute routines that should be performed in an alternating pattern two days each a week.

The weights on this plan are self-adjusting: gradually increase your weights by about 10 per cent as you gain in strength. Do not exceed the number of reps listed. For an alternative travel Bulking up workout, see pp.124–27.

repetitions (reps): the complete performance of an exercise from start position to finish position.

repetition maximum (rm): a specific number of reps for weight-related exercises, in which the muscles become so fatigued that the last few reps are hard to perform.

to failure: the number of repetitions completed until the muscles give out and fail to perform.

bulking up 3a visual overview

For alternative travel exercises, see pages 124–27

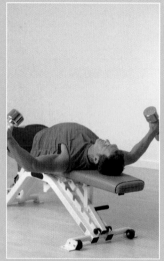

1 **pec flye** *p.93*

10 reps (3 secs per rep)

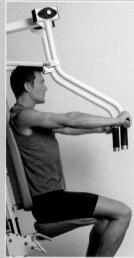

2 **chest press** *p.94*

8 reps (4 secs per rep)

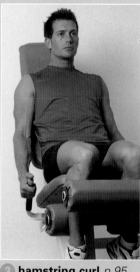

3 **hamstring curl** *p.95*

10 reps (3 secs per rep)

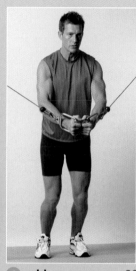

4 **cable crossover** *p.96*

8 reps (4 secs per rep)

REPEAT 1-9 x2

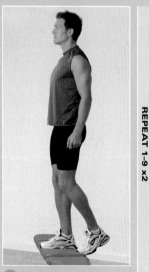

9 **bench step-up** *p.101* (each leg)

15 reps (4 secs per rep)

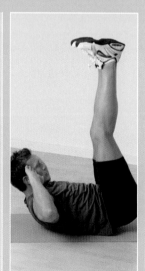

10 **advanced crunch** *p.102*

50 reps (2 secs per rep)

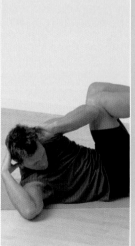

11 **alternate crossover** *p.103* (each side)

30 reps (1 sec per rep)

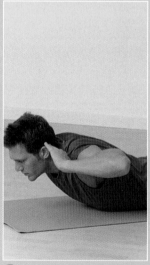

12 **back extension** *p.104*

25 reps (2 secs per rep)

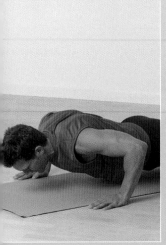

5 **press-up** *p.97*

to failure (60 secs max)

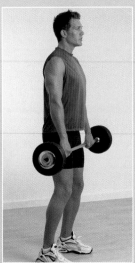

6 **dead lift** *p.98*

12 reps (3 secs per rep)

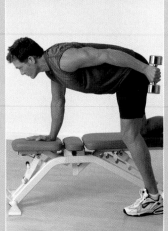

7 **tricep extension** *p.99*

10 reps (3 secs per rep)

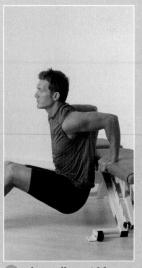

8 **tricep dip** *p.100*

to failure (45 secs max)

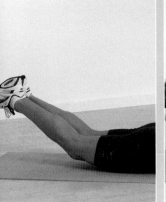

13 **reverse leg lift** *p.105*

25 reps (2 secs per rep)

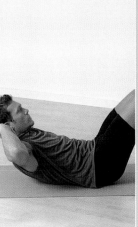

14 **basic crunch** *p.106*

50 reps (2 secs per rep)

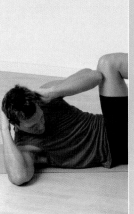

15 **isolated crossover**
p.107 (each side)

30 reps (2 secs per rep)

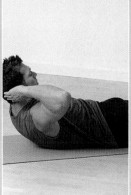

16 **straight-leg crunch**
p.106

40 reps (2 secs per rep)

REPEAT 10–16 x2

workout 3b visual overview

For alternative travel exercises, see pages 124–27

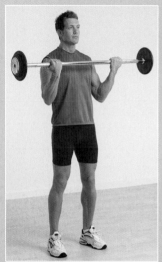

1 barbell curl *p.109*

10 reps (3 secs per rep)

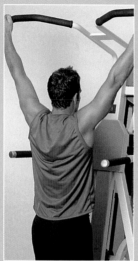

2 pull-up *p.110*

to failure (30 secs max)

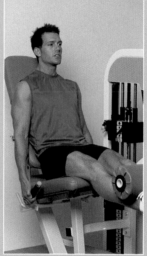

3 leg extension *p.111*

12 reps (3 secs per rep)

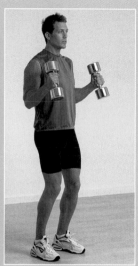

4 hammer curl *p.112*

12 reps (3 secs per rep)

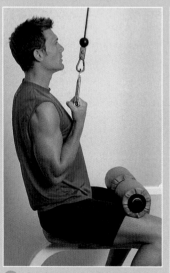

8 single-arm pull-down *p.116* (each side)

10 reps (6 secs per rep)

REPEAT 1-8 x2

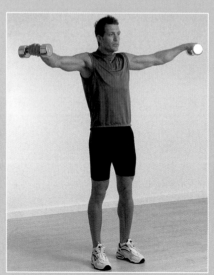

9 lateral raise *p.117*

12 reps (3 secs per rep)

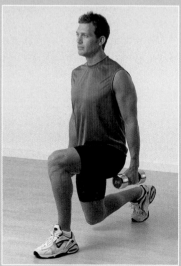

10 power lunge *p.118* (each leg)

12 reps (3 secs per rep)

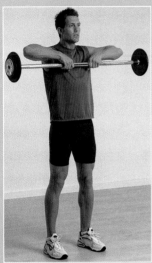
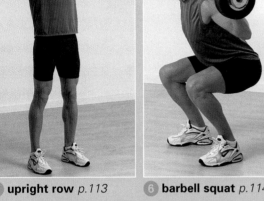
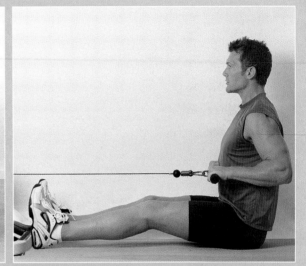

5 **upright row** *p.113*

8 reps (4 secs per rep)

6 **barbell squat** *p.114*

10 reps (3 secs per rep)

7 **seated row** *p.115*

10 reps (3 secs per rep)

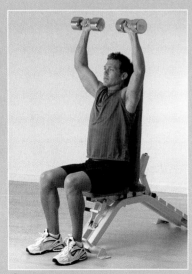
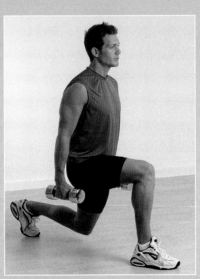
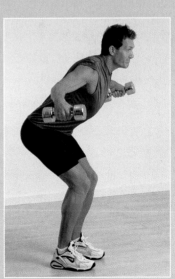

11 **shoulder press** *p.119*

10 reps (3 secs per rep)

12 **fixed lunge** *p.120*
(each leg)

12 reps (2 secs per rep)

13 **reverse flye** *p.121*

10 reps (3 secs per rep)

REPEAT 9–13 x2

workout 3a

Perform this workout two days per week in an alternating cycle with workout 3b (*pp.108–21*). In order to work the upper body muscles intensively, this workout follows a slightly different pattern of two upper body exercises and then one lower body exercise. Each exercise lists a specific number of reps to be done in a limited amount of time; once the exercise becomes easier, you should progress onto heavier weights rather than increase the number of reps.

Workout 3a targets the following muscle groups:

■ **Chest & triceps**

■ **Hamstrings & glutes**

■ **Abs & back**

 pec flye

We'll start with some isolation work on the chest muscles to give them strength and definition. Although this may be a familiar exercise, good technique is essential, so check your moves regularly.

reps	10
time	3 secs per rep

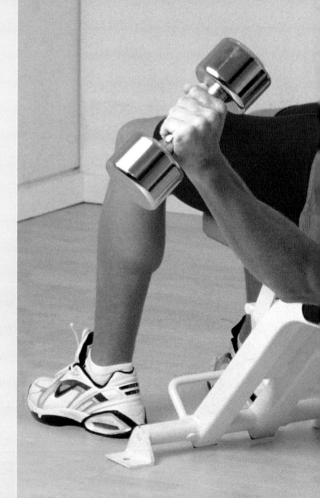

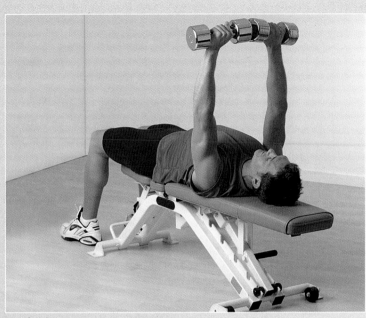

◀ step 1

- Lie back on an exercise bench
- Position feet flat on the floor or at the end of the bench
- Hold a dumbbell in each hand
- Extend arms up above chest

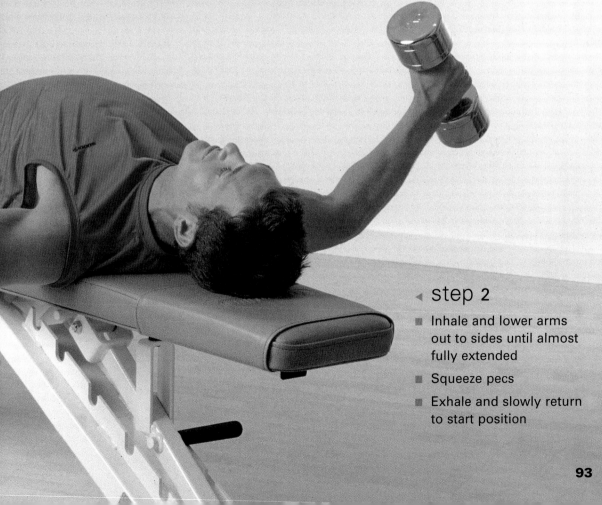

◀ step 2

- Inhale and lower arms out to sides until almost fully extended
- Squeeze pecs
- Exhale and slowly return to start position

93

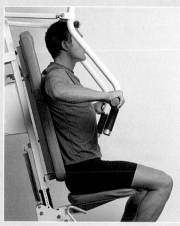

2 chest press

Get into your stride with this exercise by pushing forwards powerfully with your arms. Keep your movements controlled.

reps	8 rm
time	4 secs per rep

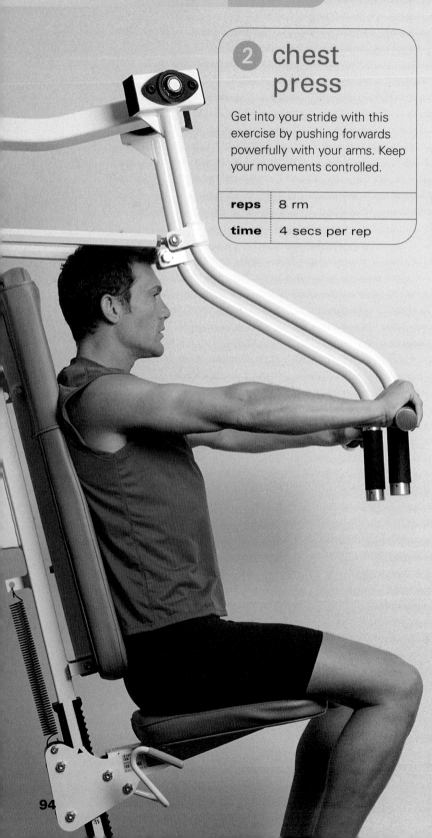

▲ step 1

- Sit at chest press machine with lower back supported
- Grasp the handles
- Bend arms until elbows are at 90°

◄ step 2

- Exhale and push forwards until arms are almost fully extended
- Keep head up and look straight ahead
- Inhale and slowly return to start position

3 hamstring curl

Move quickly over the leg curl machine to target the backs of your thighs with this lower body exercise.

reps	10 rm
time	3 secs per rep

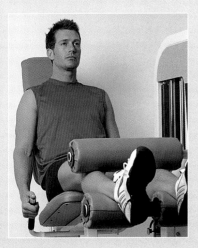

▲ step 1

- Sit at leg curl machine with lower back well supported
- Extend legs and rest ankles on roller pads
- Position large roller pad over shins

▶ step 2

- Tighten abs and exhale
- Push your heels towards your buttocks
- Inhale and return to start position

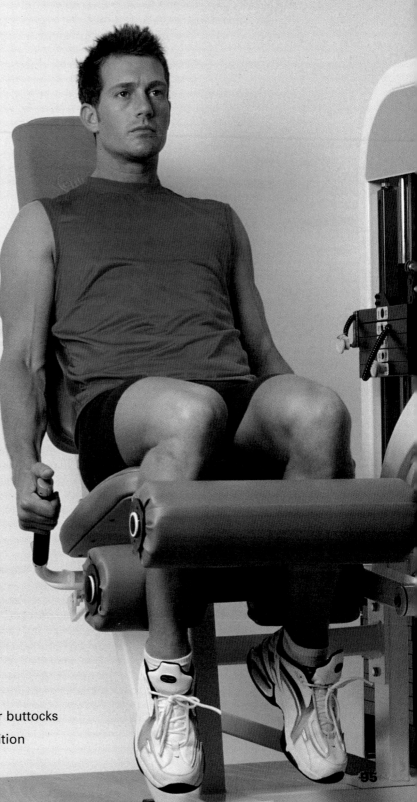

95

4 cable crossover

If a cable crossover machine is not available in your gym, exercise your arms separately on a single cable machine.

reps	8 rm
time	4 secs per rep

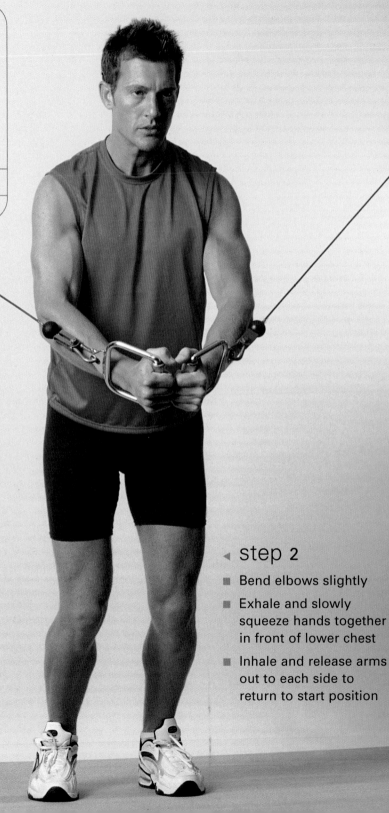

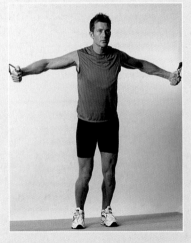

▲ step 1

- Stand at a cable machine, equidistant from the pulley handles
- Grasp each handle so that palms face inwards
- Lean forwards a little and bend knees slightly

◄ step 2

- Bend elbows slightly
- Exhale and slowly squeeze hands together in front of lower chest
- Inhale and release arms out to each side to return to start position

(5) press-up

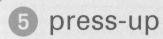

A simple but effective exercise: the press-up uses the weight of your own body as resistance so that you quickly build up strength in your pecs, deltoids, and triceps. Keep your fingers facing forwards, your body weight over your hands, your back flat, and your abs tight as you work.

reps	to failure
time	60 secs maximum

▼ step 1

- Balance on toes and hands
- Position hands just wider than shoulder-width apart
- Straighten your back and legs

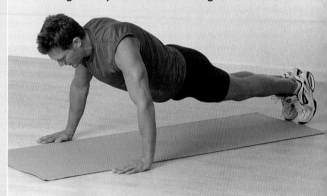

▼ step 2

- Inhale and lower torso down
- Bend elbows out at 90°
- Exhale and push back up to start position

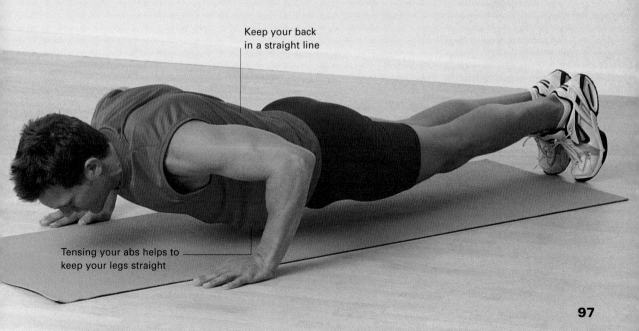

Keep your back in a straight line

Tensing your abs helps to keep your legs straight

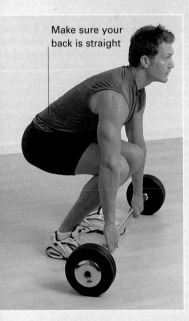

Make sure your back is straight

6 dead lift

This barbell exercise targets your pecs, deltoids, biceps, and triceps in one big hit. You'll soon see the difference.

reps	12 rm
time	3 secs per rep

▲ step 1

- Position a barbell on the ground
- Place feet hip-width apart behind barbell
- Bend knees 90°
- Lean body forwards
- Grasp the barbell with your hands shoulder-width apart
- Look straight ahead

◄ step 2

- Exhale and slowly stand up
- Keep your arms and back straight
- Keep the barbell close to the body
- Pull your shoulder blades back
- Inhale and slowly return to start position

⑦ tricep extension

Some isolation work for your triceps; keep your abs tight and your back straight. Do all the reps on one arm, then change sides.

reps	10 rm
time	3 secs per rep

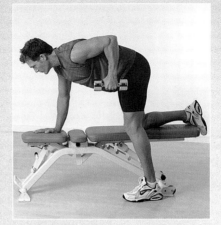

◄ step 1

- Rest right hand and knee on an exercise bench
- Keep left foot on the floor
- Hold a dumbbell in your left hand
- Lift arm and bend elbow until it is at 90° to the floor

◄ step 2

- Keep upper arm and elbow still
- Exhale and extend lower arm
- Flex your tricep
- Inhale and lower down to start position

Your upper arm should remain parallel to the floor

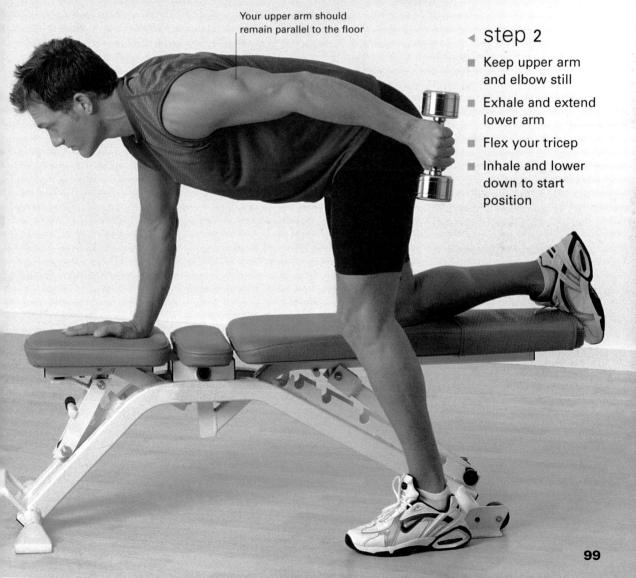

step 1

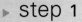

- Hold onto the edge of an exercise bench with palms facing backwards
- Position feet away from the bench
- Straighten arms

8 tricep dip

Your arms should really be feeling it by now, so this may seem like a killer exercise. It works so well because you lift against the resistance of your own body weight.

reps	to failure
time	45 secs maximum

step 2

- Inhale and lower torso down until elbows are at 90°
- Exhale and slowly push back up to start position
- Don't lock your arms at the top of the movement

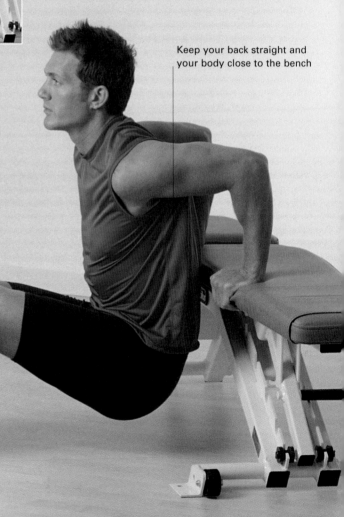

Keep your back straight and your body close to the bench

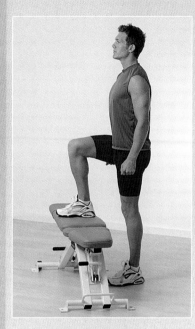

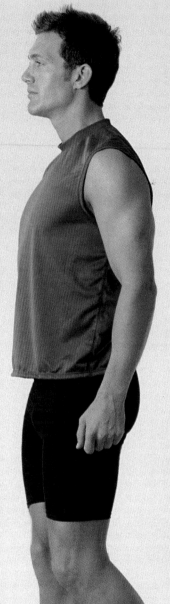

9 bench step-up

Step-ups not only build strength in your leg muscles (particularly your glutes), they also raise your heart rate. Perform 15 step-ups with your right foot leading, then swap legs and complete 15 more reps with your left leg leading.

reps	15 each leg
time	4 secs per rep

▲ step 1

- Stand facing the exercise bench
- Keep your back straight
- Relax head and neck and align with spine
- Rest right foot on bench

◀ step 2

- Exhale and step up with your whole foot flat on the bench
- Step up with the left foot
- Inhale and step down, right foot first
- Repeat immediately, without pause

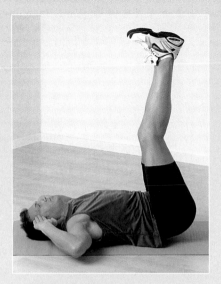

⑩ advanced crunch

This superior abdominal exercise will work your abs hard. It may seem tough to begin with, but you'll soon build core strength to cope with this intense blitzing of your abs.

reps	50
time	2 secs per rep

▲ step 1

- Lie on your back on a mat
- Raise legs in the air
- Place hands at the sides of your head
- Tighten abs

◂ step 2

- Exhale and lift your shoulder blades off the floor
- Curl shoulders forwards
- Keep lower back on the floor
- Inhale and lower down to start position

Keep your chin up

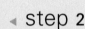

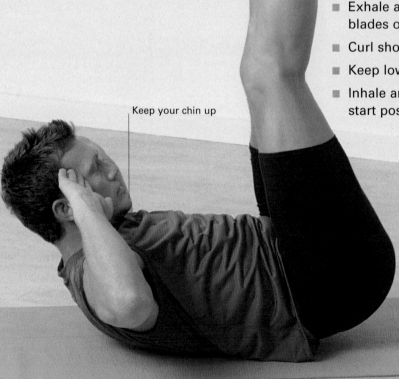

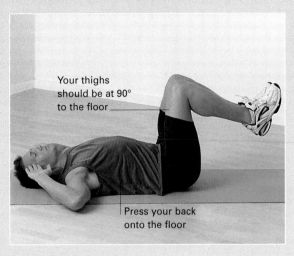

Your thighs should be at 90° to the floor

Press your back onto the floor

⑪ alternate crossover

Your abs and obliques will get an extra tough workout from this exercise: keep them tight throughout so that you maintain your balance while your legs are in the air. Alternate your movements for a total of 60 reps.

reps	30 each side
time	1 sec per rep

▲ step 1

- Lie on your back on a mat
- Raise legs in the air
- Bend your knees
- Place hands at the sides of your head
- Tighten abs

▼ step 2

- Exhale and raise one shoulder and elbow
- Point your left elbow towards your right knee
- Return to start position
- Repeat on alternate side

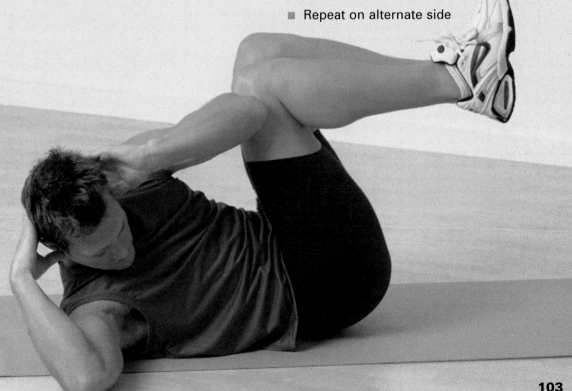

back extension

This is an excellent exercise for building strength in your lower back muscles, which should enable you to protect your whole back effectively and improve your posture.

reps	25
time	2 secs per rep

▾ **step 1**

- Lie on your front on a mat
- Place hands at the sides of your head
- Tighten abs and point toes

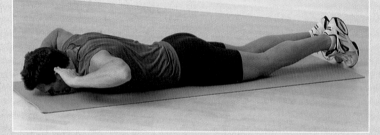

▾ **step 2**

- Exhale and raise your head and upper body
- Keep hips and toes pressed onto the floor
- Hold for one second
- Inhale and lower back down to start position

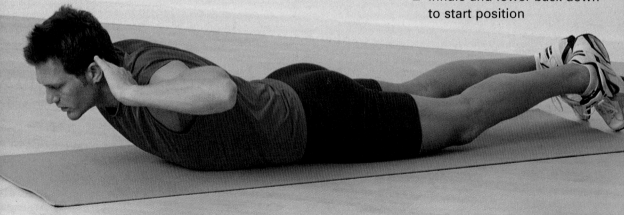

step 1

- Lie on your front on a mat
- Rest forehead on hands
- Press palms onto the floor
- Tighten abs

Keep your chest on the floor at all times

13 reverse leg lift

This lower body exercise is great for strengthening the lower back and building the glutes. The better you control your upward movement, the more effectively you'll work your muscles.

reps	25
time	2 secs per rep

step 2

- Exhale and lift both legs in air, as high as possible
- Raise knees off floor and keep legs as straight as you can
- Keep knees and heels together
- Inhale and lower down to start position

basic crunch & straight-leg crunch

The basic crunch, in which your feet remain on the floor, is a simple sit-up, but done properly it is a powerfully effective workout for your abs, and will help to sculpt your waistline. Keeping your legs straight for the straight-leg crunch encourages your abs to work harder at the base.

basic crunch		straight-leg crunch	
reps	50	reps	40
time	2 secs per rep	time	2 secs per rep

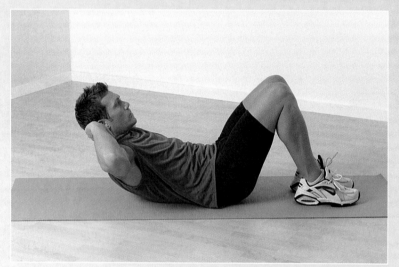

◄ basic crunch

- Lie on your back on a mat
- Bend knees and place feet hip-width apart on floor
- Place hands at the sides of your head
- Tighten abs
- Exhale and raise shoulders and chest upwards
- Inhale and lower down to start position

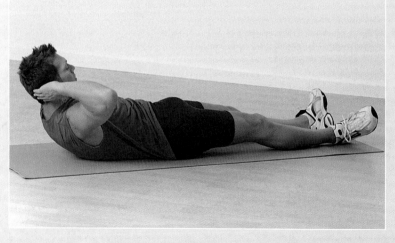

◄ straight-leg crunch

- Lie on your back on a mat
- Extend legs
- Press lower back onto floor
- Place hands at the sides of your head
- Tighten abs
- Exhale and raise shoulders and chest upwards
- Inhale and lower down to start position

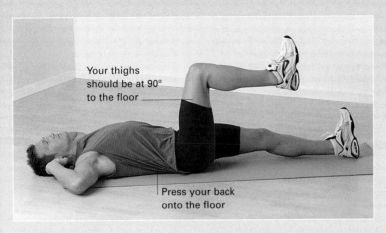

Your thighs should be at 90° to the floor

Press your back onto the floor

⑮ isolated crossover

Isolating the work you do on the obliques creates impressive muscle definition through the lower torso. Do all the reps on one side, then swap sides.

reps	30 each side
time	2 secs per rep

▲ step 1

- Lie on your back on a mat, legs extended
- Raise right leg in the air and bend knee 90°
- Place hands at the sides of your head
- Tighten abs

▼ step 2

- Exhale and twist from the waist across to the right
- Raise left elbow to elevated right knee
- Inhale and lower down to start position

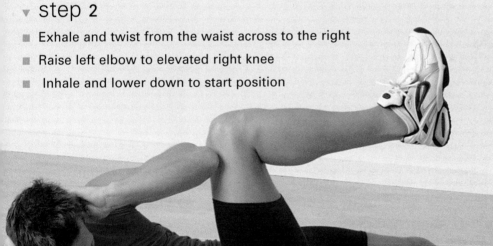

workout 3b

Perform this workout two days per week in an alternating cycle with workout 3a *(pp.92–107)*. In order to work the upper body muscles intensively, this workout follows a slightly different pattern of two upper body exercises and then one lower body exercise. Each exercise lists a specific number of reps to be done in a limited amount of time; once the exercise becomes easier, you should progress onto heavier weights rather than increase the number of reps.

Workout 3b targets the following muscle groups:

- **Biceps**
- **Back**
- **Quads**
- **Shoulders**

 barbell curl

This intensive exercise gives great definition and strength to the biceps. Flex your muscles as you lift the barbell up to shoulder height to really feel the bicep muscles working hard. Keep your back straight and abs tight throughout.

reps	10
time	3 secs per rep

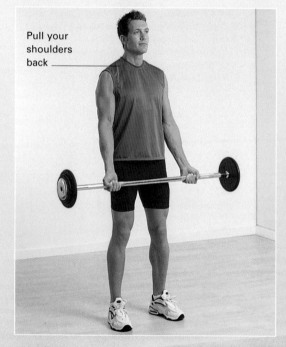

Pull your shoulders back

▲ **step 1**

- Stand with feet hip-width apart
- Keep knees slightly bent
- Hold a barbell in front of the body
- Your palms should face outwards

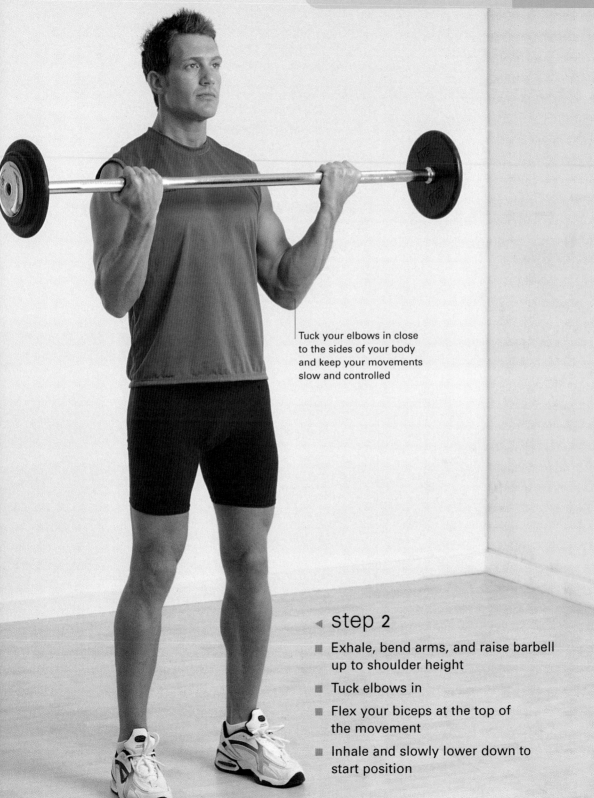

Tuck your elbows in close to the sides of your body and keep your movements slow and controlled

◄ **step 2**

■ Exhale, bend arms, and raise barbell up to shoulder height

■ Tuck elbows in

■ Flex your biceps at the top of the movement

■ Inhale and slowly lower down to start position

2 pull-up

Push yourself to the limit on the pull-up, which works the large back muscles. As you gain strength, move off the machine to a full unassisted pull-up on a bar.

reps	to failure
time	30 secs maximum

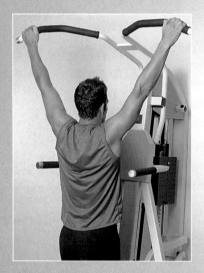

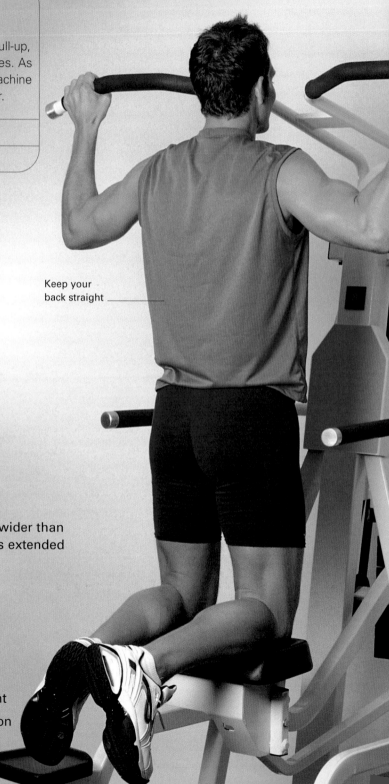

Keep your back straight

▲ step 1

- Kneel up on pull-up machine
- Hold the bar with both hands wider than shoulder-width apart and arms extended
- Tighten abs

▶ step 2

- Exhale and pull yourself up
- Stop when eyes are level with the bar
- Make sure your back is straight
- Inhale and lower to start position

③ leg extension

This is an intense workout for the quads, and your muscles will soon react to the overload generated by this exercise. Don't let the weights drop completely in between lifts.

reps	12 rm
time	4 secs per rep

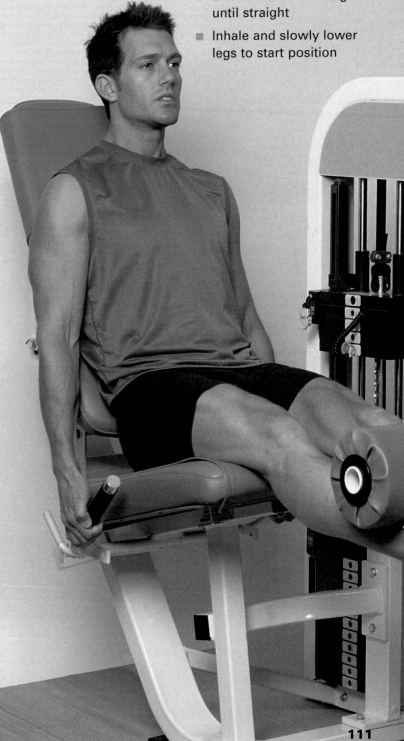

▼ step 2

- Exhale and extend legs until straight
- Inhale and slowly lower legs to start position

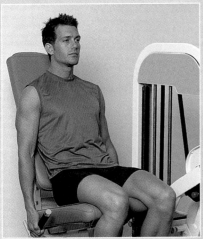

▲ step 1

- Sit at leg extension machine with lower back supported
- Hook ankles behind the roller pad so that knees are at 90°
- Tighten abs and point toes

④ hammer curl

This variation on the bicep curl is a great way of working the outer sections of the biceps to give greater muscle mass.

reps	12 rm
time	3 secs per rep

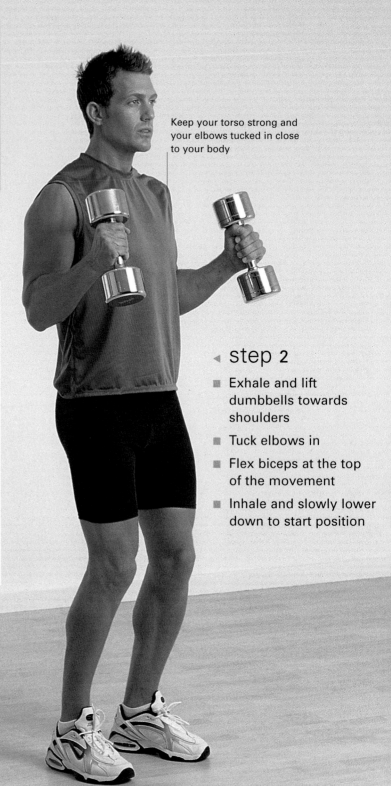

Keep your torso strong and your elbows tucked in close to your body

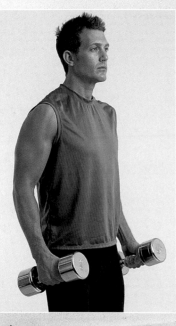

▲ step 1

- Hold dumbbells at sides with palms facing in towards you
- Stand with feet hip-width apart
- Bend knees slightly

◀ step 2

- Exhale and lift dumbbells towards shoulders
- Tuck elbows in
- Flex biceps at the top of the movement
- Inhale and slowly lower down to start position

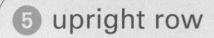

⑤ upright row

This exercise will target the shoulder muscles and biceps to create incredible definition.

reps	8 rm
time	4 secs per rep

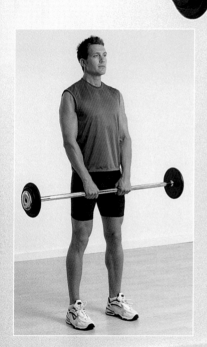

◀ **step 2**

- Exhale and draw barbell up to chest height

- Lead with your elbows

- Inhale and slowly lower barbell down to start position

▲ **step 1**

- Hold a barbell in front of you, palms facing in towards you

- Stand with feet hip-width apart

- Straighten your back

113

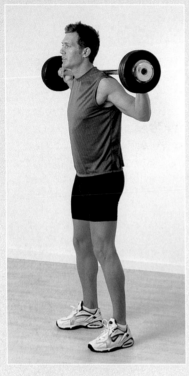

⑥ barbell squat

You will really work your thighs and buttocks with this exercise: using a barbell will intensify the effort required by your leg muscles to work against such heavy resistance.

reps	10 rm
time	3 secs per rep

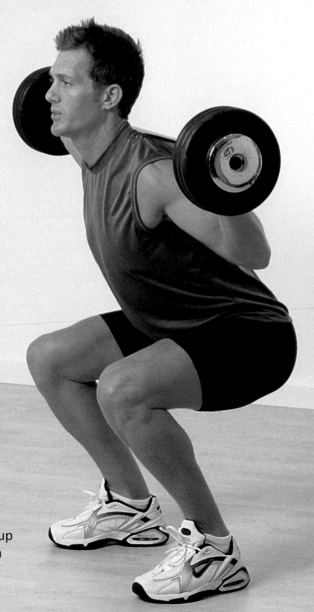

▲ step 1

- Stand with feet hip-width apart
- Place a barbell across shoulder blades
- Straighten your back
- Tighten abs

▶ step 2

- Inhale and bend knees until thighs are parallel to the floor
- Keep back straight
- Exhale and slowly push back up through heels to start position

▼ step 1

- Sit on floor facing a cable machine
- Extend legs almost fully and rest heels against machine
- Hold bar with both hands

Keep your back straight

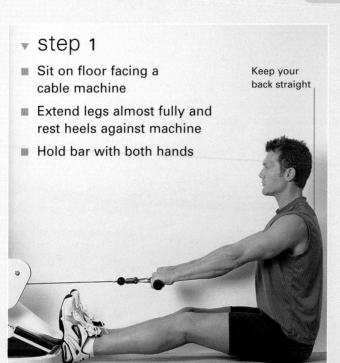

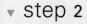

⑦ seated row

Move on quickly to the cable machine to target the muscles of your upper middle back. Keep your elbows tucked into your sides as you pull back and forth with strong movements.

reps	10 rm
time	3 secs per rep

▼ step 2

- Exhale and pull bar in close to lower chest
- Keep elbows tucked in
- Hold for one second
- Inhale and return to start position

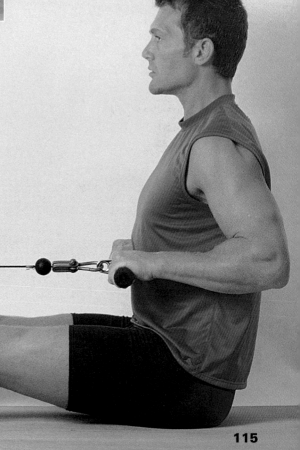

⑧ single-arm pull-down

This tough exercise requires you to use a wide array of muscle groups to stabilize your body while your biceps and back muscles work intensively. Avoid leaning backwards as you pull down.

reps	10 rm each side
time	6 secs per rep

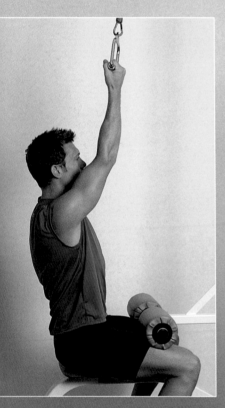

◀ **step 2**

- Exhale and pull handle down to chest level
- Keep your body still
- Keep your hand and elbow towards the outside, rather than in front, of your body
- Inhale and release up to start position

▲ **step 1**

- Sit facing a lat pull-down machine
- Hold handle with your palm facing towards you
- Extend arm almost fully above head
- Keep your back straight

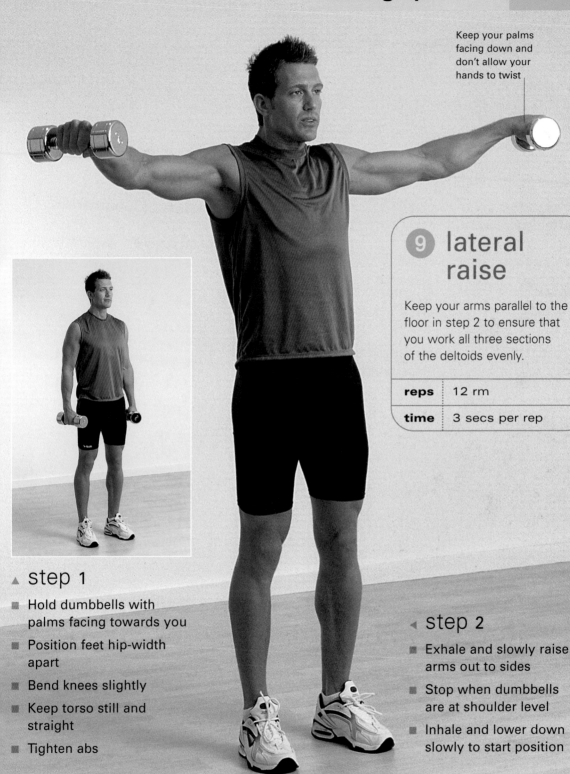

Keep your palms facing down and don't allow your hands to twist

⑨ lateral raise

Keep your arms parallel to the floor in step 2 to ensure that you work all three sections of the deltoids evenly.

reps	12 rm
time	3 secs per rep

▲ step 1

- Hold dumbbells with palms facing towards you
- Position feet hip-width apart
- Bend knees slightly
- Keep torso still and straight
- Tighten abs

◄ step 2

- Exhale and slowly raise arms out to sides
- Stop when dumbbells are at shoulder level
- Inhale and lower down slowly to start position

117

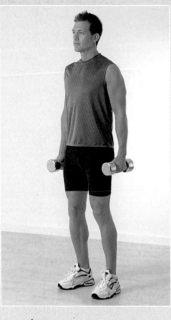

10 power lunge

This version of lungeing helps you to build powerful, sculpted leg muscles, particularly the glutes and adductor muscles. Spring back up to start position if you want to increase the intensity of the movement. Alternate your legs for each rep.

reps	12 each leg
time	3 secs per rep

▲ step 1

- Hold a dumbbell in each hand, palms facing in towards you
- Stand with feet hip-width apart
- Keep your head up
- Stride forwards with one leg

◄ step 2

- Inhale and bend back knee down towards floor
- Bring front knee directly over front foot
- Shift body weight onto heel of front foot
- Exhale and spring back up to start position

⑪ shoulder press

Sitting to perform this exercise will support your torso and concentrate the workload onto the deltoid muscles; stand up if you want to give your triceps more of a challenge. Keep the momentum going and focus on making your movements strong.

reps	10 rm
time	3 secs per rep

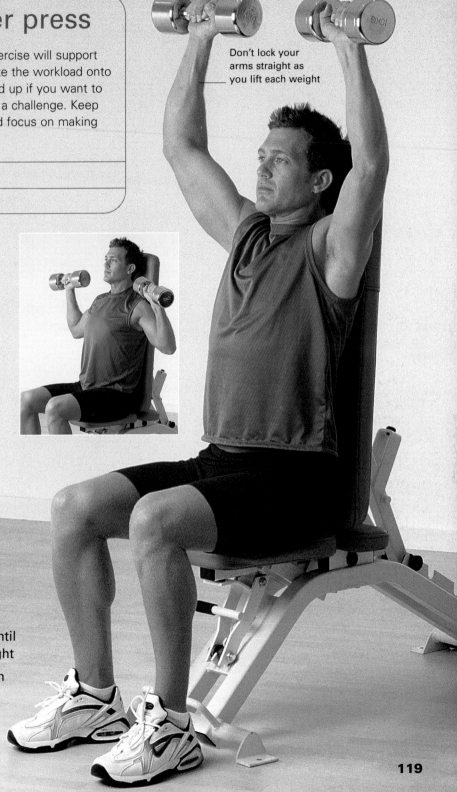

Don't lock your arms straight as you lift each weight

▶ step 1

- Hold a dumbbell in each hand
- Sit on exercise bench and ensure that lower back is supported
- Hold elbows out to sides
- Keep arms bent at 90°
- Tighten abs

▶ step 2

- Exhale and raise arms above head
- Press dumbbells up until arms are almost straight
- Inhale and lower down to start position

119

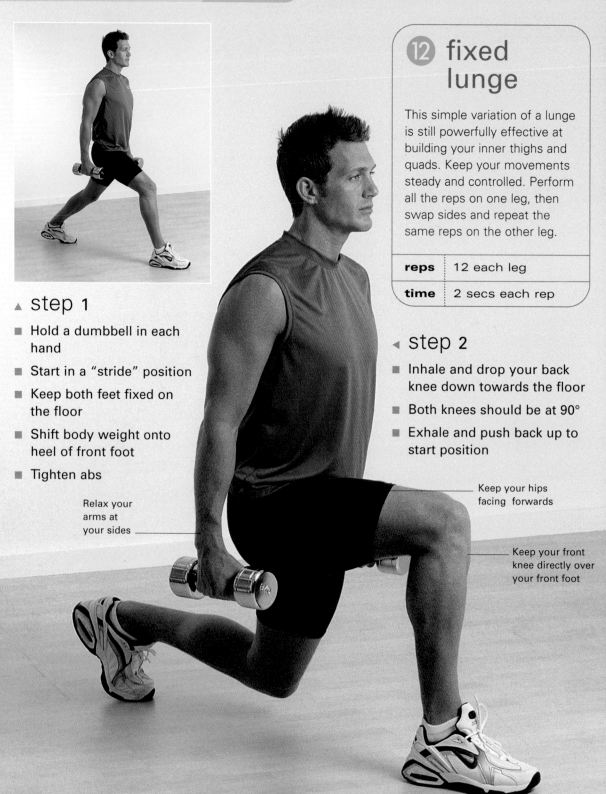

⑫ fixed lunge

This simple variation of a lunge is still powerfully effective at building your inner thighs and quads. Keep your movements steady and controlled. Perform all the reps on one leg, then swap sides and repeat the same reps on the other leg.

reps	12 each leg
time	2 secs each rep

▲ step 1

- Hold a dumbbell in each hand
- Start in a "stride" position
- Keep both feet fixed on the floor
- Shift body weight onto heel of front foot
- Tighten abs

Relax your arms at your sides

◂ step 2

- Inhale and drop your back knee down towards the floor
- Both knees should be at 90°
- Exhale and push back up to start position

Keep your hips facing forwards

Keep your front knee directly over your front foot

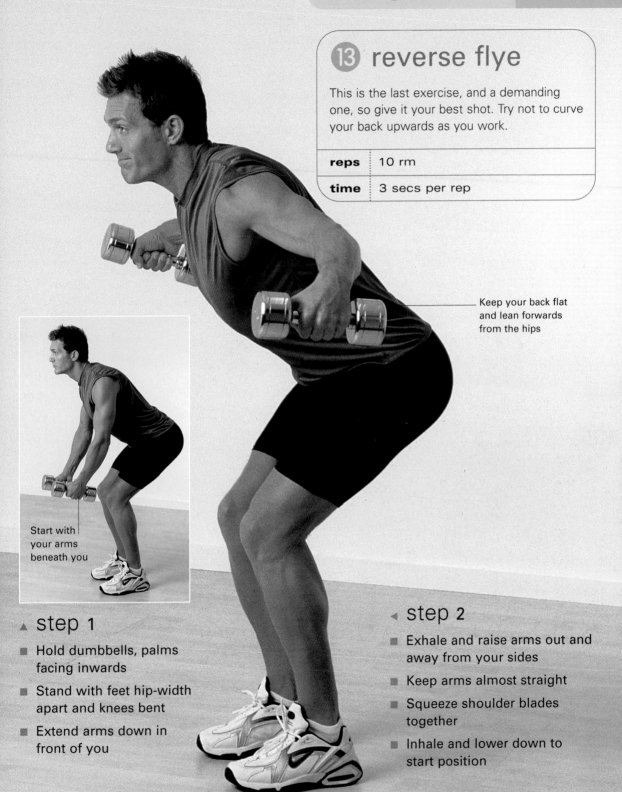

⑬ reverse flye

This is the last exercise, and a demanding one, so give it your best shot. Try not to curve your back upwards as you work.

reps	10 rm
time	3 secs per rep

Keep your back flat and lean forwards from the hips

Start with your arms beneath you

▲ step 1

- Hold dumbbells, palms facing inwards
- Stand with feet hip-width apart and knees bent
- Extend arms down in front of you

◄ step 2

- Exhale and raise arms out and away from your sides
- Keep arms almost straight
- Squeeze shoulder blades together
- Inhale and lower down to start position

121

questions & answers

You have to be committed to working out if you want to get great results on the Bulking up programme. Having said that, there are other important aspects of your health to consider, such as eating a balanced diet, if you want to achieve optimum muscle mass and strength.

Q I have heard that that you should eat lots of protein after a workout. Is this true, and if so, why?

a Protein is the main source of amino acids, a group of nutrients required by the body in order to repair and maintain internal organs and body tissue. When you work your body hard to see improvements in muscle mass, it is essential that you supply it with enough amino acids for post-exercise repair (p.86). However, the amount of protein that you require is not a massive amount, and it equates to eating no more than a tin of tuna a day. If you are performing four workouts a week and you rest properly in between sessions, you won't need to eat extra protein. Just ensure that there is a good level of protein in your normal diet.

Q What percentage of my diet should contain carbohydrates, proteins, and fats?

a Your body needs the right kind of food in order to function efficiently, digest food, filter impurities, fight disease, and provide you with enough energy to be active. A healthy diet must include all the nutrients the body requires to maintain this equilibrium. Firstly, you need an abundant supply of carbohydrate, the prime supplier of energy to the body. Certain carbohydrates, known as low-glycaemic carbohydrates, contain energy that is released to the body over a longer period of time, and, therefore, helps to maintain your energy levels more consistently. These carbohydrates tend to be the unrefined, wholesome carbs (rather than heavily processed "white" carbs), and include foods such as brown rice, wholewheat pasta, wholemeal bread, quinoa, apples, pears, chick-peas, beans, peppers, and carrots. These healthy carbs should make up about 55–60 per cent of your diet.

Protein is the nutrient responsible for helping the body heal and repair itself, and maintain skin, tissues, and strong muscles (see left). Protein is found in meat, fish, nuts, dairy products, and some grains. Eat a wide variety of proteins to make up 25–30 per cent of your diet.

The other elements that are essential to a healthy diet are fat and fibre. Your diet should be higher in essential fats and as low as possible in saturated fats. Saturated fats play no useful role in the body, and can be harmful to the heart in large quantities. Essential fats are required by the body for a variety of functions, including the production of energy, improving the quality of skin and hair, and for weight management. Essential fats are found in foods such as olives, oily fish, nuts and cold-pressed oils. Fats should make up no more than 20 per cent of your diet, with 95 per cent of that figure consisting of essential fats. The basic role of fibre is to help the body, and in particular the digestive system, cleanse

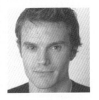

Your **body** needs the **right kind** of **food** to **function** properly and provide you with enough **energy**

itself. Without fibre, all other functions in the body are inhibited. Foods rich in fibre include fresh and dried fruit, vegetables, oats, brown rice, and whole wheat products.

If I miss a workout one week, should I do five workouts the next week to make up for it?

Provided that this is the only approach you are taking, and that you only do it now and again, yes. If you are tempted to do just one workout one week and seven the following week, then I would say no. However, minor alterations like this are fine if you lead a busy lifestyle, and if it will help you to stay on course to achieve your personal fitness goals, then, yes, you can do it occasionally.

If I want to concentrate on working just one particular part of my body, will the Bulking up programme enable me to do that?

The fitness programmes in this book are designed to achieve different goals for different people. The beauty of a PHA workout is that it both affects the size and shape of your muscles, and improves the cardiovascular conditioning of your body. The fact that I have applied these PHA principles to every programme means that I want you to concentrate

on working your whole body rather than particular areas. It is my view that any workout should aim to have overall benefits on the body. Use this approach for the Bulking up programme, and the results will be far more effective than trying to target individual areas.

If I have a muscle injury, can I keep working other areas of the body while I rest the muscle?

Depending upon where the injury is, it should be possible for you to keep exercising. Provided that you are able to perform exercises that have no direct impact on the damaged area, you should not be in danger of causing any further problems – and it is entirely possible that you may actually recover more quickly as a result of exercising.

The most difficult exercises to perform when injured are the dynamic exercises, because they have an impact on a large number of muscle groups. Dynamic exercises usually affect such a wide variety of muscle groups that, if you perform these while injured, further damage may be likely. In general, aerobic exercises work all areas of the body, whereas resistance exercises tend to work isolated muscle groups. It is worth seeking medical advice from your doctor first if you are unsure of the extent of your injury, to check that you don't cause long-lasting damage to your body if you continue to exercise.

bulking up travel alternative

If you have any doubts how you'll gain muscle size while you are travelling, you can rest assured that there are ways of exercising that will, at worst, prevent you going backwards and, at best, provide an effective alternative workout that maintains your current fitness levels. As always, focus on technique, keep up the momentum, and make each movement powerful to overload the muscles.

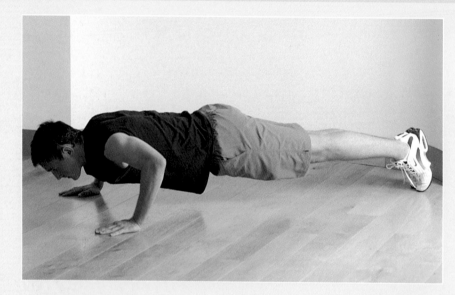

1 press-up

- Balance on toes and hands
- Position hands just wider than shoulder-width apart
- Inhale and lower torso down until elbows are at 90°
- Exhale and push up to start position
- Reps = 25–30

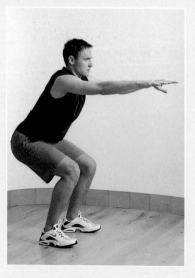

3 squat

- Stand with feet hip-width apart
- Tighten abs and inhale
- Bend knees 90° until thighs are parallel with floor
- Keep back upright, arms out in front for balance
- Exhale and push up through heels
- Reps = 30–40

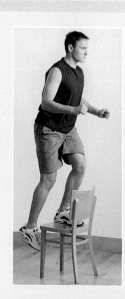

4 step-up

- Stand facing a chair
- Keep back straight
- Exhale and step up with left foot flat on the chair
- Step up with right foot
- Inhale and step down, one foot at a time
- Reps = 25 each leg

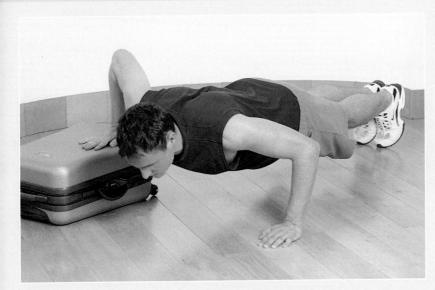

② press-up with one hand elevated

- Place right hand on a step or hard suitcase, and left hand on the floor
- Balance on toes and hands
- Hands should be just wider than shoulder-width apart
- Inhale and lower torso until left elbow is at 90°
- Exhale and push up to start position
- Reps = 20 each side

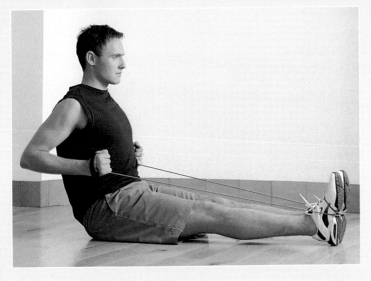

⑤ seated row

- Sit upright on the floor with legs straight
- Wrap exertube around feet until it feels taut
- Grasp handles and wrap excess tube around hands until taut
- Exhale and pull handles into side of lower torso
- Keep elbows tucked in
- Inhale and return to start position
- Reps = 20

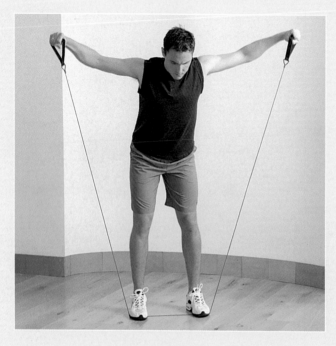

6 reverse flye

- Stand on exertube, feet hip-width apart
- Grasp handles with palms facing towards your sides
- Lean forwards slightly with straight back
- Exhale and raise arms out and away from sides
- Lift handles up to shoulder height, keeping arms almost straight
- Inhale and lower down to start position
- Reps = 25

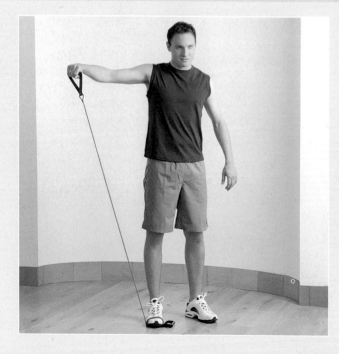

8 single-arm lateral raise

- Stand with feet hip-width apart
- Wrap end of exertube around right foot
- Grasp handle in right hand, palm facing towards your sides, and tighten abs
- Exhale and slowly lift right arm out to shoulder height
- Inhale and lower down to start position
- Reps = 20 each side

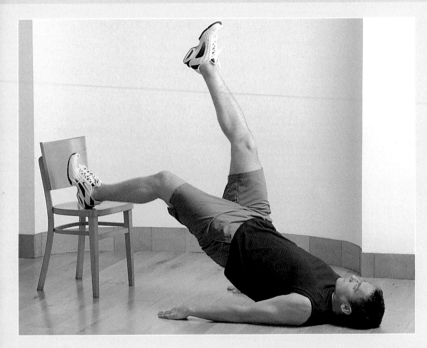

7 single-leg body lift

- Lie on back on the floor, arms at sides
- Rest left foot on a chair
- Raise right leg in the air
- Exhale and lift pelvis until torso is in a straight line
- Inhale and lower down to start position
- Reps = 25 each side

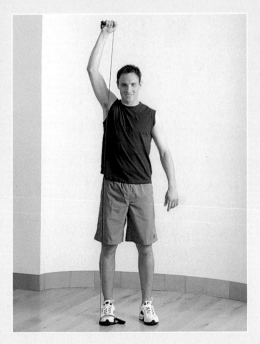

9 single-arm shoulder press

- Stand with feet hip-width apart
- Wrap end of exertube around right foot
- Grasp remaining handle in right hand
- Bend elbow and position hand at shoulder height
- Exhale and raise arm straight up
- Avoid locking your arm straight
- Inhale and lower to start position
- Reps = 20 each side

bulking up training log

When you are looking to increase muscle size, you can't afford to waste a workout. So it's important that you record all the weights you use to help you try to achieve more with each successive workout.

workout 3a

exercise	date: weight	date: weight
pec flye set 1		
chest press set 1		
hamstring curl set 1		
cable crossover set 1		
press-up set 1		
dead lift set 1		
tricep extension set 1		
tricep dip set 1		
bench step-up set 1		
pec flye set 2		
chest press set 2		
hamstring curl set 2		
cable crossover set 2		
press-up set 2		
dead lift set 2		
tricep extension set 2		
tricep dip set 2		
bench step-up set 2		
pec flye set 3		
chest press set 3		
hamstring curl set 3		
cable crossover set 3		
press-up set 3		
dead lift set 3		

exercise (continued)	weight	weight
tricep extension set 3		
tricep dip set 3		
bench step-up set 3		
advanced crunch set 1		
alternate crossover set 1		
back extension set 1		
reverse leg lift set 1		
basic crunch set 1		
isolated crossover set 1		
straight-leg crunch set 1		
advanced crunch set 2		
alternate crossover set 2		
back extension set 2		
reverse leg lift set 2		
basic crunch set 2		
isolated crossover set 2		
straight-leg crunch set 2		
advanced crunch set 3		
alternate crossover set 3		
back extension set 3		
reverse leg lift set 3		
basic crunch set 3		
isolated crossover set 3		
straight-leg crunch set 3		

Use **large loadings** of weight
to create **fantastic muscle mass**

workout 3b	date:	date:
exercise	**weight**	**weight**
barbell curl set 1		
pull-up set 1		
leg extension set 1		
hammer curl set 1		
upright row set 1		
barbell squat set 1		
seated row set 1		
single-arm pull-down set 1		
barbell curl set 2		
pull-up set 2		
leg extension set 2		
hammer curl set 2		
upright row set 2		
barbell squat set 2		
seated row set 2		
single-arm pull-down set 2		
barbell curl set 3		
pull-up set 3		
leg extension set 3		
hammer curl set 3		
upright row set 3		
barbell squat set 3		

exercise (continued)	**weight**	**weight**
seated row set 3		
single-arm pull-down set 3		
lateral raise set 1		
power lunge set 1		
shoulder press set 1		
fixed lunge set 1		
reverse flye set 1		
lateral raise set 2		
power lunge set 2		
shoulder press set 2		
fixed lunge set 2		
reverse flye set 2		
lateral raise set 3		
power lunge set 3		
shoulder press set 3		
fixed lunge set 3		
reverse flye set 3		

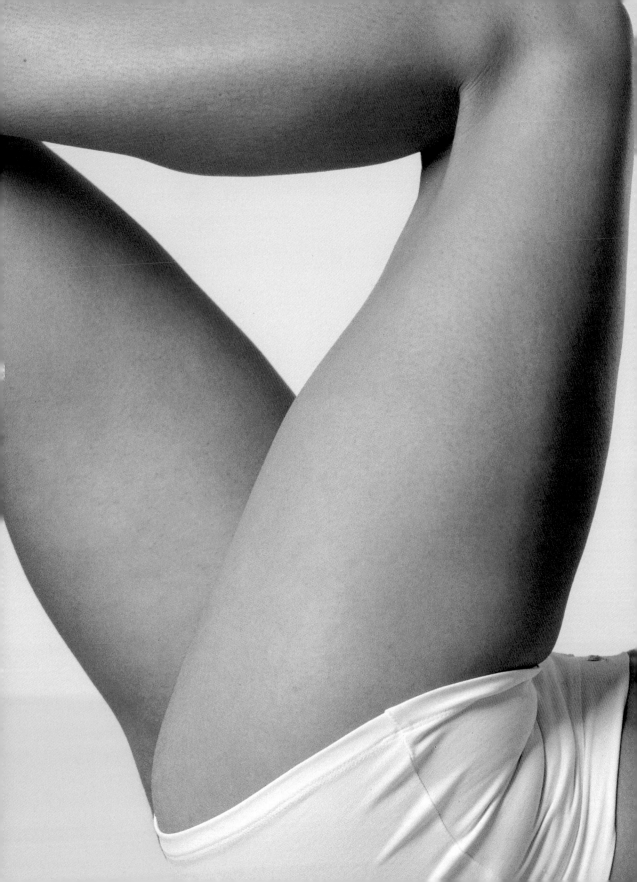

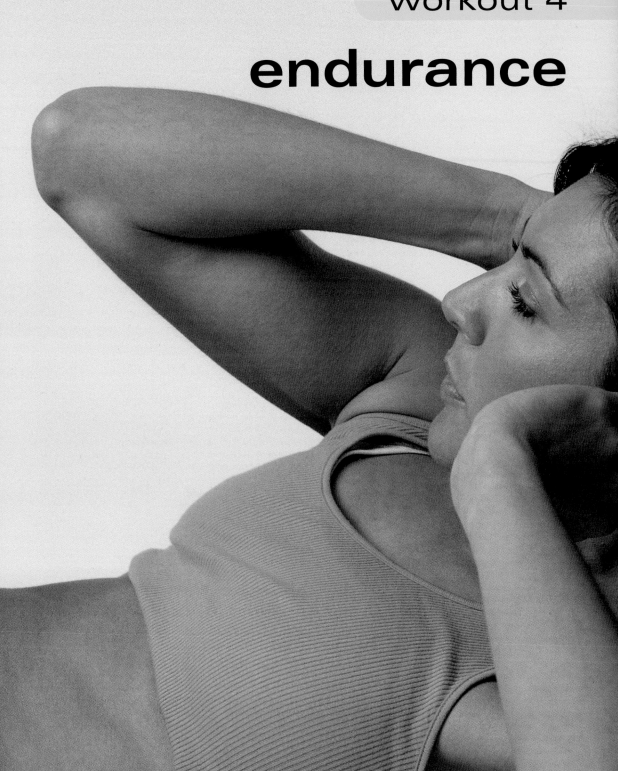

endurance

endurance programme

Why do an Endurance programme? Well, this type of training will generally make you feel much fitter so that you are able to cope with a range of other exercises that you may want to participate in. If you run, play any multi-sprint sports, or do triathlons, this programme will make you truly fit.

It is often the case that if you play a sport, and perhaps complement it with resistance work to increase your strength, you may be training with weights in a way that is unsuitable because you don't want to inhibit your agility. This Endurance programme, however, will give you speed, strength and stamina. It's one that I have successfully used with premiership footballers: the workout allows them to maintain a high degree of mobility, which

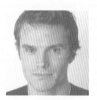

You'll be **surprised** how far you can **push yourself** under pressure

they depend on, but it also gives them additional strength, power and, importantly, stability, which reduces the risk of injury when they play football.

Programme structure
This 45-minute PHA workout uses time rather than repetitions as the main mechanism for working individual body areas. You'll also be using weights to build muscular endurance, not muscle mass.

We'll begin with the largest dynamic compound exercises (when muscle groups work in conjunction with one another), and spend a while focusing on each area of the body, so you'll be doing as many reps as you can in the limited time allowed.

By starting with these major muscle areas, we'll be able to test your muscular endurance thoroughly. In between each set of exercises, you'll be further challenged by short periods of time on either a rowing machine or a cross-trainer. This aerobic input will fatigue the body even more, and put you into a physical state that will force your body to adapt its muscular endurance levels. As the workout progresses, the emphasis moves from dynamic compound exercises to isolation exercises (when just one muscle group is used). This is because we'll be focusing on the smaller muscle groups to produce intense local muscular fatigue in areas such as the biceps, triceps, and glutes.

Pushing through your limits
The key to this workout is to ensure that you work to a very high level during your aerobic time on the rower or cross-trainer to reach a point of fatigue. Once you reach that point, really push yourself to allow your body to overload (p.76).

You'll be surprised how far you can push yourself under pressure; in many cases, people don't work as hard as they think. A recently published research paper in the US found that out of a group of people tested on a specific workout, 47 per cent felt they reached a moderate level of intensity, when actually only 11 per cent did. That small percentage felt that they pushed themselves to a vigorous level, but according to their heart rates only two per cent did!

So, even when you feel fatigued, you can still push yourself harder. The gains you can make on this PHA Endurance programme are, therefore, incredible, and very safe.

workout 4 – four times a week for six weeks

warm-up: rower or cross-trainer (build to 8–10 RPE) 10 minutes

exercise	level 1	level 2	level 3
pull-up	30 secs	45 secs	60 secs
jump squat	30 secs	45 secs	60 secs
press-up	30 secs	45 secs	60 secs
fixed lunge	30 secs each leg	45 secs each leg	60 secs each leg
advanced crunch	30 secs	45 secs	60 secs

repeat set above, then move on to set below

rower or cross-trainer (8–9 RPE) 3 minutes

lateral pull-down	30 secs	45 secs	60 secs
seated squat	30 secs	45 secs	60 secs
tricep dip	30 secs	45 secs	60 secs
bench step-up	30 secs each leg	45 secs each leg	60 secs each leg
advanced crossover	30 secs	45 secs	60 secs

repeat set above, then move on to set below

rower or cross-trainer (8–9 RPE) 3 minutes

alternate bicep curl	30 secs	45 secs	60 secs
leg extension	30 secs	45 secs	60 secs
tricep push-down	30 secs	45 secs	60 secs
hamstring curl	30 secs	45 secs	60 secs
reverse curl	30 secs	45 secs	60 secs

repeat set above, then move on to final exercise below

rower or cross-trainer (8–9 RPE) 3 minutes, then (6–7 RPE) 1 minute, then (very easy pace) 1 minute

cool-down (*pp.20–23*)

The aim here is to develop muscular endurance rather than pure strength. Select a weight that allows you to perform 15–20 reps for each exercise. Begin at level 1: complete one rep every two seconds for 30 seconds. When you can manage this for every exercise, increase the time – not the weight – to 45 seconds, level 2. Once you reach level 3 and complete the circuit working for 60 seconds on every exercise, increase the weights. For alternative Endurance travel workout, see pages 154–55.

rate of perceived exertion (RPE): a self-grading system of how hard you think that you are working, on a scale from 0 (lying down) to 10, the maximum effort that you can possibly achieve (*see also* rate of exertion, *p.19*).

endurance visual overview

For alternative travel exercises, see pages 154–55

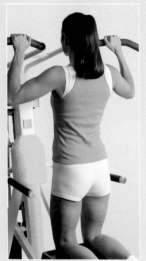

1 pull-up *p.136*

30 secs 45 secs 60 secs

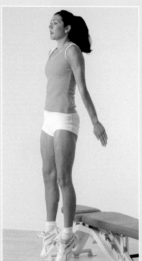

2 jump squat *p.137*

30 secs 45 secs 60 secs

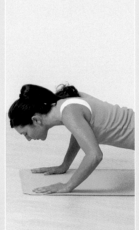

3 press-up *p.138*

30 secs 45 secs 60 secs

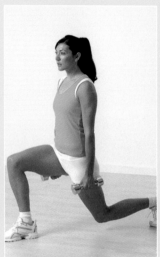

4 fixed lunge *p.139*
(each leg)

30 secs 45 secs 60 secs

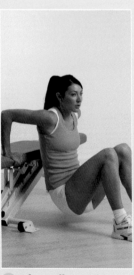

9 tricep dip *p.144*

30 secs 45 secs 60 secs

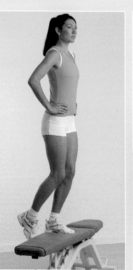

10 bench step-up *p.145*
(each leg)

30 secs 45 secs 60 secs

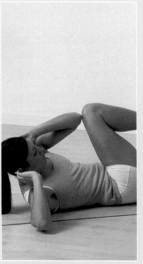

11 advanced crossover *p.146*

30 secs 45 secs 60 secs

REPEAT 7–11, THEN 6, THEN MOVE ON TO 12

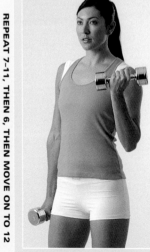

12 alternate bicep curl *p.147*

30 secs 45 secs 60 secs

key　| level 1 | level 2 | level 3 |

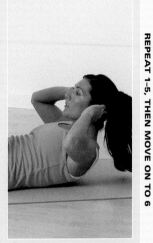

REPEAT 1–5, THEN MOVE ON TO 6

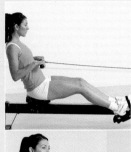

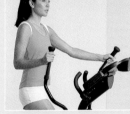

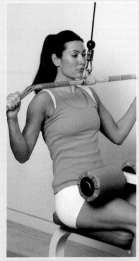

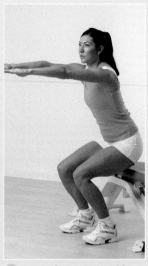

5 **advanced crunch** *p.140*

30 secs　45 secs　60 secs

6 **rower or cross-trainer** *p.141*

3 mins　3 mins　3 mins

7 **lateral pull-down** *p.142*

30 secs　45 secs　60 secs

8 **seated squat** *p.143*

30 secs　45 secs　60 secs

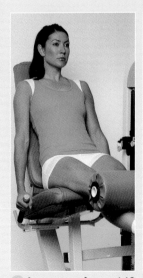

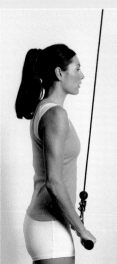

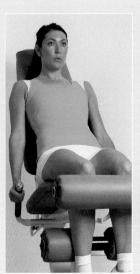

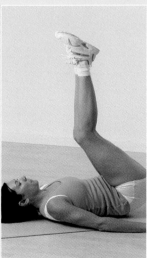

REPEAT 12–16, THEN 6, THEN REPEAT ×2 MINS SLOW

13 **leg extension** *p.148*

30 secs　45 secs　60 secs

14 **tricep push-down** *p.149*

30 secs　45 secs　60 secs

15 **hamstring curl** *p.150*

30 secs　45 secs　60 secs

16 **reverse curl** *p.151*

30 secs　45 secs　60 secs

135

pull-up

Your lats will be seriously tested with this first exercise. Even though you will be using a weight-assisted pull-up machine, try to lift the equivalent of your body weight.

level 1	30 secs
level 2	45 secs
level 3	60 secs

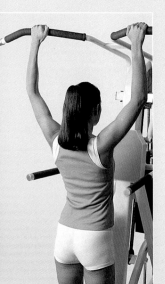

◄ step 1

- Kneel up at a pull-up machine
- Hold bar with both hands wider than shoulder-width apart and arms almost straight

Keep your body as straight as possible _____

▶ step 2

- Exhale and pull yourself up
- Stop when your eyes are level with the bar
- Inhale and slowly lower yourself down to start position

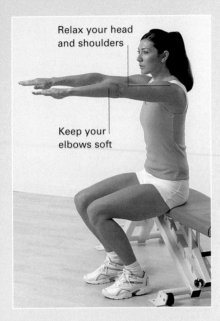

Relax your head and shoulders

Keep your elbows soft

▲ step 1

- Stand in front of an exercise bench
- Position feet hip-width apart
- Extend arms out in front of you
- Squat down on the edge of the exercise bench

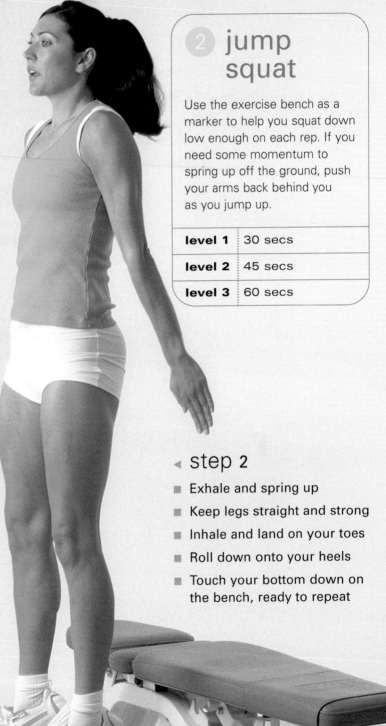

② jump squat

Use the exercise bench as a marker to help you squat down low enough on each rep. If you need some momentum to spring up off the ground, push your arms back behind you as you jump up.

level 1	30 secs
level 2	45 secs
level 3	60 secs

◄ step 2

- Exhale and spring up
- Keep legs straight and strong
- Inhale and land on your toes
- Roll down onto your heels
- Touch your bottom down on the bench, ready to repeat

press-up

It may be a simple and familiar exercise, but the press-up is a tough resistance workout for your pecs, deltoids, and triceps so that they'll give you that extra bit of strength when you need it most. Keep your fingers facing forwards, your body weight over your hands, your back flat, and your abs tight. Try a modified technique (*p.30*) if you find the full press-up hard going.

level 1	30 secs
level 2	45 secs
level 3	60 secs

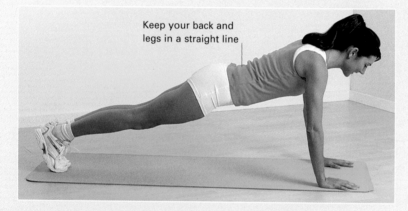

Keep your back and legs in a straight line

◄ ## step 1

- Position hands just wider than shoulder-width apart
- Balance on toes and hands
- Straighten your back

▼ ## step 2

- Inhale and lower torso down
- Bend elbows out at 90°
- Exhale and push back up to start position

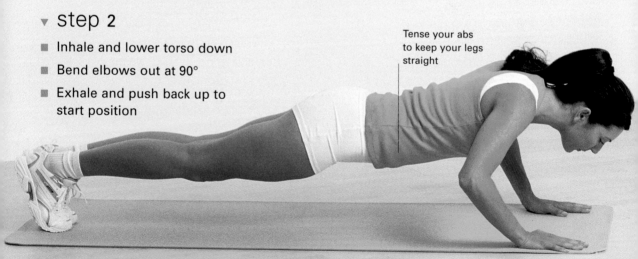

Tense your abs to keep your legs straight

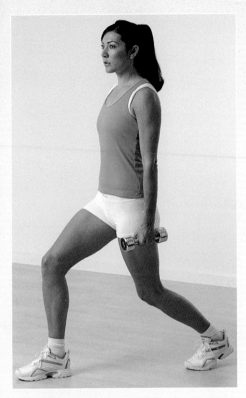

▲ step 1

- Hold a dumbbell in each hand
- Start in a "stride" position
- Keep both feet fixed on the floor
- Shift body weight onto heel of front foot
- Tighten abs

▶ step 2

- Inhale and drop back knee towards the floor
- Both knees should be at 90°
- Keep front knee directly over front foot
- Exhale and push up to start position

4 fixed lunge

Move swiftly on to this classic lower body exercise. All the major leg muscles are targeted, so you should build power quickly in your legs. Repeat on one leg for 30 seconds, then swap sides for another 30 seconds.

level 1	30 secs each leg
level 2	45 secs each leg
level 3	60 secs each leg

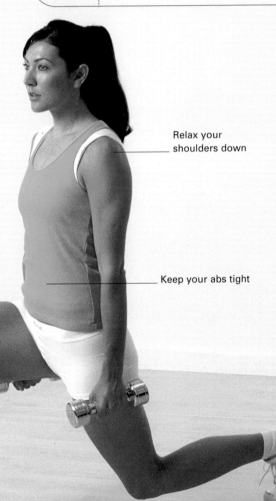

Relax your shoulders down

Keep your abs tight

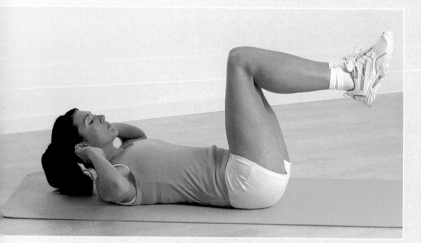

⑤ advanced crunch

This version of the crunch maintains a constant pressure on the abs, which intensifies its effectiveness. Keep your legs still for the best results.

level 1	30 secs
level 2	45 secs
level 3	60 secs

▲ step 1

- Lie on your back on a mat
- Raise feet off the floor
- Bend knees 90°
- Place hands at the sides of your head
- Tighten abs

▼ step 2

- Exhale and lift shoulder blades off floor
- Curl shoulders forwards
- Keep lower back on floor
- Inhale and lower down to start position

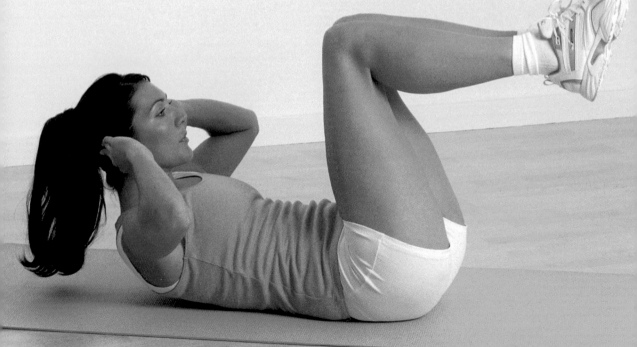

⑥ rower or cross-trainer

Rower Rowing is an excellent aerobic exercise that works your upper and lower body at the same time. It requires the correct technique and some coordination to get the maximum benefit. The "recoil" action should take twice the amount of time as the "pull" action.

Cross-trainer This machine targets a wide range of muscles: it works more lower body muscles than any other aerobic machine in the gym, and it works them evenly. The result is that you can quickly raise your heart rate and concentrate on building your stamina.

level 1	3 mins
level 2	3 mins
level 3	3 mins

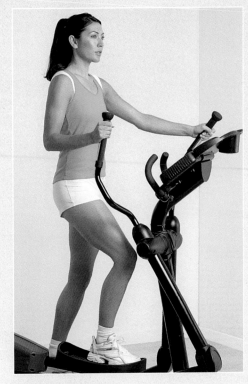

▲ cross-trainer

- Stand tall on the machine
- Tighten abs
- Press backwards through your feet by "clawing" at the pedals
- Work arms and legs at same rate

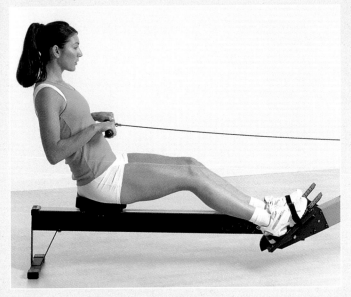

◂ rower

- Start with knees bent and arms extended
- Exhale, pull bar into lower chest and push back with legs
- Lean back slightly
- Tuck elbows into sides
- Inhale and return to start position

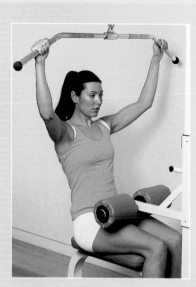

◄ **step 1**

- Sit at a lat pull-down machine
- Hold the bar firmly
- Position hands slightly wider than shoulder-width apart
- Lean back slightly
- Tighten abs

⑦ lateral pull-down

This machine works the large muscles of the back: the latissimus dorsi, or lats, and the rhomboids. Keep your back straight as you pull the bar down. Each repetition should take two to three seconds.

level 1	30 secs
level 2	45 secs
level 3	60 secs

▶ **step 2**

- Exhale and pull down
- Bring elbows in close to body
- Squeeze the base of the shoulder blades together
- Inhale and return to start position

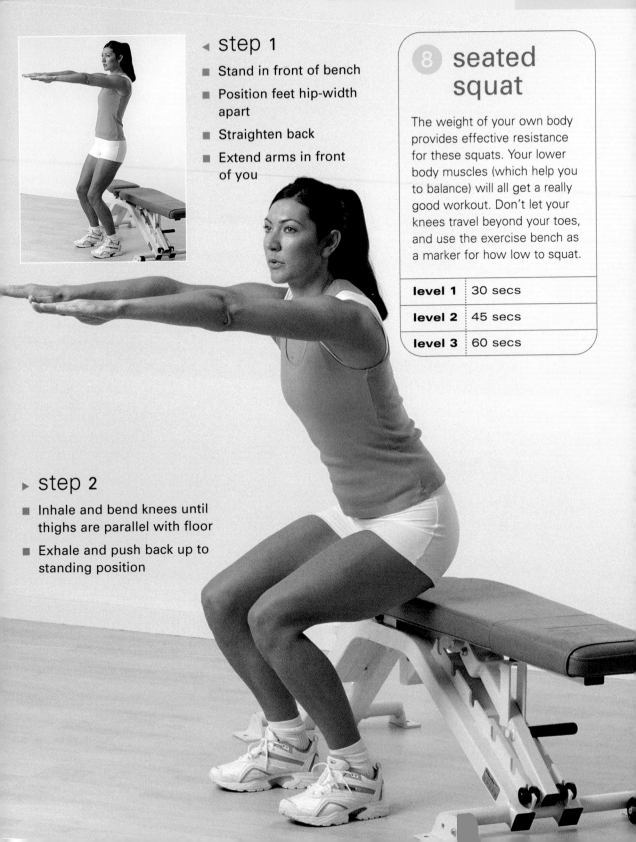

◂ step 1

- Stand in front of bench
- Position feet hip-width apart
- Straighten back
- Extend arms in front of you

⑧ seated squat

The weight of your own body provides effective resistance for these squats. Your lower body muscles (which help you to balance) will all get a really good workout. Don't let your knees travel beyond your toes, and use the exercise bench as a marker for how low to squat.

level 1	30 secs
level 2	45 secs
level 3	60 secs

▸ step 2

- Inhale and bend knees until thighs are parallel with floor
- Exhale and push back up to standing position

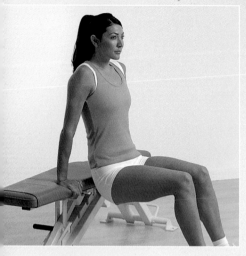

9 tricep dip

Quickly transfer onto an exercise bench for this exercise. Make the exercise more difficult by moving your feet further away from you.

level 1	30 secs
level 2	45 secs
level 3	60 secs

▲ step 1

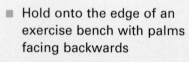

- Hold onto the edge of an exercise bench with palms facing backwards
- Position feet away from the bench
- Straighten arms

Keep your back straight

▼ step 2

- Inhale and lower torso down until elbows are at 90°
- Exhale and push back up
- Don't lock your arms at the top of the movement

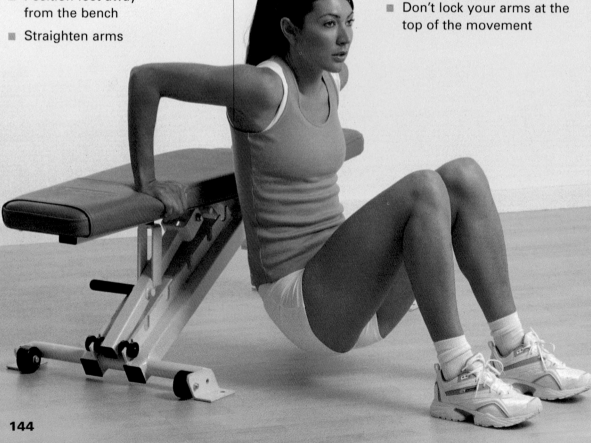

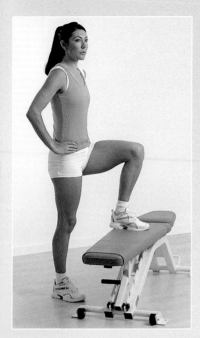

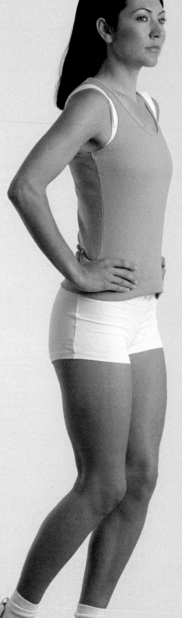

10 bench step-up

Keep up the pace and do these step-ups as powerfully as you can to raise your heart rate and build stamina in the legs. Swap your lead foot halfway through.

level 1	30 secs each leg
level 2	45 secs each leg
level 3	60 secs each leg

▲ step 1

- ■ Stand facing an exercise bench
- ■ Keep your back straight
- ■ Relax head and neck and align with spine
- ■ Place left foot flat on bench

◄ step 2

- ■ Exhale and step onto bench
- ■ Place your whole foot flat on the bench
- ■ Step up with the right foot
- ■ Inhale and step down, left foot first
- ■ Repeat immediately, without pause

145

▼ step 1

- Lie on your back on a mat
- Position feet flat on floor, bend knees and place hands at sides of your head
- Raise shoulder blades off the floor
- Tighten abs and inhale

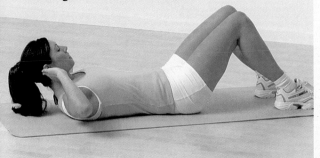

⑪ advanced crossover

This exercise challenges your obliques. Rotate through the body, reaching towards the knee to really work your waist. Focus on keeping your abs tight.

level 1	30 secs
level 2	45 secs
level 3	60 secs

▼ step 2

- Lift extended left leg off floor and bend right knee
- Exhale and raise left elbow to right knee
- Twist from waist across to the right, then inhale and lower down
- Repeat on alternate sides without stopping

Your raised elbow should touch your elevated knee

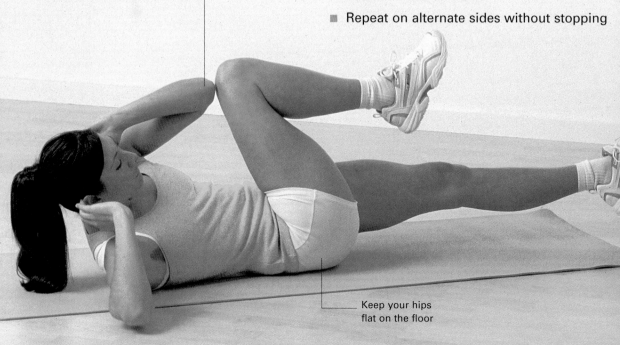

Keep your hips flat on the floor

alternate bicep curl

This intensive exercise strengthens the upper arms. Flex your biceps as you lift each dumbbell to your shoulder so that you maximize the effectiveness of the exercise.

level 1	30 secs
level 2	45 secs
level 3	60 secs

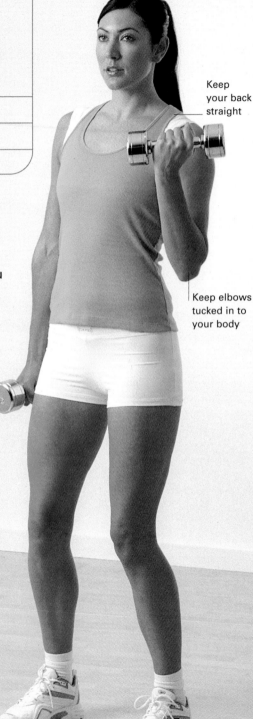

Keep your back straight

Keep elbows tucked in to your body

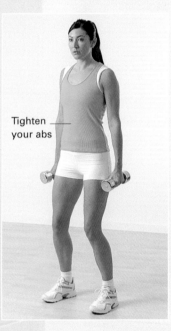

Tighten your abs

◄ step 1

- Hold a dumbbell in each hand, palms facing in towards you
- Stand with feet hip-width apart
- Bend knees slightly
- Relax arms at sides
- Tuck elbows in

► step 2

- Exhale, bend left arm and raise dumbbell to shoulder
- Turn dumbbell out towards shoulder at top of movement and flex bicep
- Inhale and return to start position
- Repeat on alternate sides without stopping

⑬ leg extension

This exercise effectively works the quads, the large muscle group at the front of each thigh. Keep your toes pointed at all times to avoid bulking the muscles. Control your movements throughout, and don't let the weights drop completely in between each lift.

level 1	30 secs
level 2	45 secs
level 3	60 secs

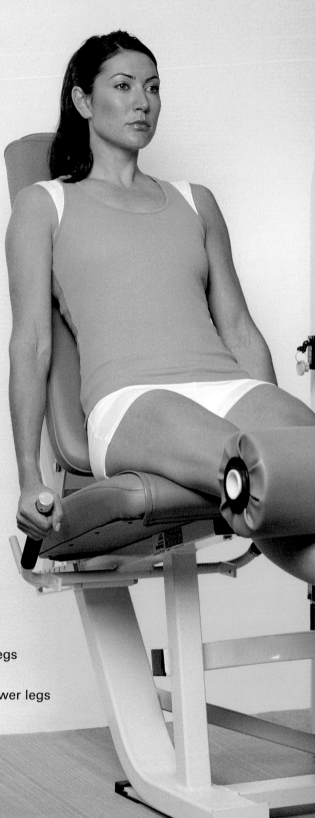

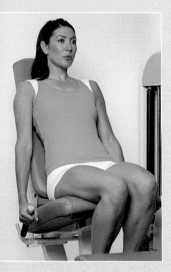

◂ step 1

- Sit at leg extension machine and ensure that lower back is supported

- Hook ankles behind the roller pad so that knees are at 90°

- Tighten abs and point toes

▸ step 2

- Exhale and extend legs until straight

- Inhale and slowly lower legs to start position

⑭ tricep push-down

By now your whole body is probably fatigued. This exercise gives your other muscles a brief rest, and shifts attention onto the small but important tricep muscle at the back of each arm.

level 1	30 secs
level 2	45 secs
level 3	60 secs

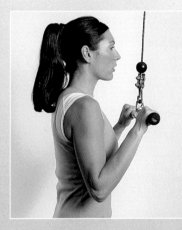

▲ step 1

■ Stand facing a lat pull-down machine with your back straight

■ Grasp handle at shoulder height and tuck elbows in

▶ step 2

■ Exhale and push handle down to hips

■ Keep elbows tucked into sides

■ Inhale and release up to start position

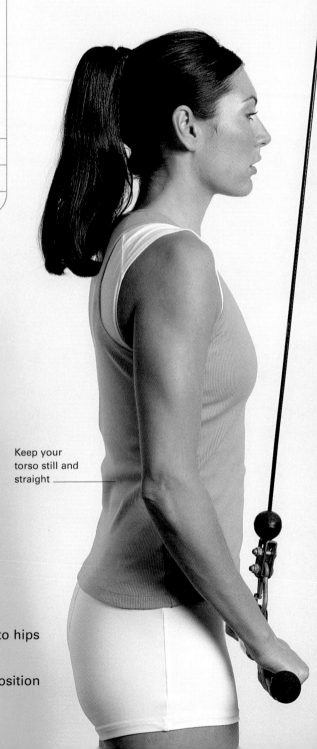

Keep your torso still and straight

149

⑮ hamstring curl

One last hamstring exercise to give you the power to keep going and provide that extra burst of strength, which is so important in many sports. If this feels like a real test of your stamina, concentrate on working against the clock.

level 1	30 secs
level 2	45 secs
level 3	60 secs

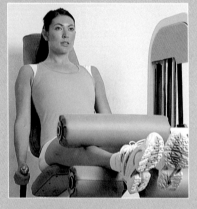

▲ step 1

- Sit at leg curl machine with lower back supported and legs extended
- Rest ankles on roller pads
- Position large roller pad over shins

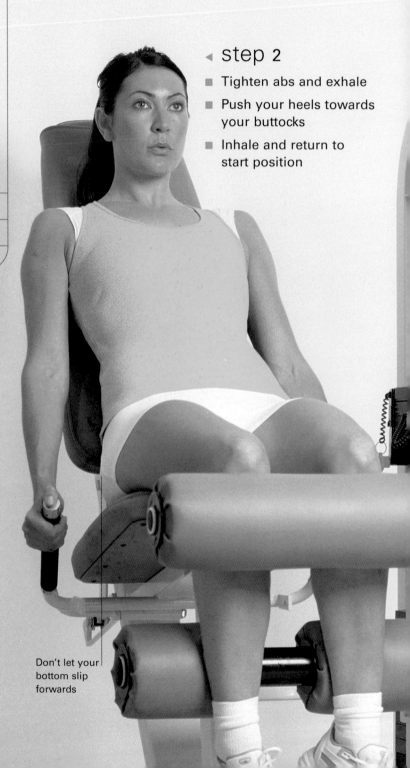

◄ step 2

- Tighten abs and exhale
- Push your heels towards your buttocks
- Inhale and return to start position

Don't let your bottom slip forwards

▼ step 1

- Lie on your back on a mat
- Press palms onto floor
- Raise legs straight in the air

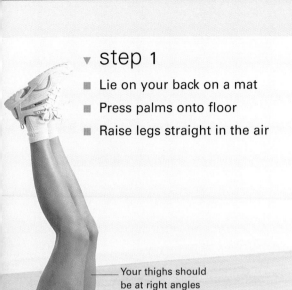

Your thighs should be at right angles to your body

reverse curl

This may feel like a bit of a killer to end the workout, but tough it out and you'll soon have fantastically strong abs. Keep your head and shoulders flat on the floor throughout.

level 1	30 secs
level 2	45 secs
level 3	60 secs

▼ step 2

- Tighten lower abs and exhale
- Curl legs and pelvis towards chest
- Inhale and lower down slowly to start position

questions & answers

It's easy to get into a routine and think that the longer you spend following a programme, the more likely it is that you will reach your optimum performance level. Instead, you need to keep re-assessing how effective your training is, and how best to achieve your fitness goals.

Q **Just how long can I carry on doing the same PHA workout for? Will I keep getting great results?**

a You should update and modify your training routine on a session-by-session basis. If the weight you have chosen to perform a number of reps on the Endurance programme starts to feel easy to work against, you should move up a level to increase the time limit and number of reps, until eventually you reach level 3. After that, consider increasing the weight you use. As a general rule, a 10 per cent increase in weight is usually about right. Re-assess your goals and how your training is progressing every six to eight weeks: in that time your body will have become used to the routine, and won't have to make the same physiological adaptations as it did to start with. This could inhibit your physical achievements, so you may want to move onto another PHA programme and find fresh motivation.

Q **Can a person exercise too much? How do I know when I'm overdoing it?**

a It is possible to exercise too much, and it's easy to end up putting the effort into exercise without reaping any of the rewards that are normally associated with it. The main problem with over-exercising is

that you don't give your muscles enough time to recover in between workouts. The whole aim of exercising is to push the body hard and break down the muscle fibres, so that during the post-exercise recovery period they repair themselves to become stronger (*p.76, p.86*). Thus, over a period of time the body actually becomes stronger and stronger. This recovery period usually takes about 48 hours, but without sufficient recovery time this repair stage can never be properly completed by the body.

While this doesn't mean that you can't exercise every day, it does mean that the exercise plan you follow must be designed in such a way that the muscles you use on one day are not used in the same way the following day. The programmes in this book – with the exception of the Bulking up programme – are designed to be performed on a day on/day off rota to give you maximum benefit.

Q **What is the best kind of food for me to eat before and after a PHA workout?**

a If you are eating a healthy, balanced diet that includes carbohydrates and proteins (*p.122*), and drinking plenty of water, you should have enough energy stored within the body beforehand to get you through every workout in this book. If, however, you are working out at the end of the day and you

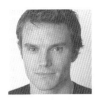

Re-assess your fitness goals and how your training is progressing every six to eight weeks

regularly feel lethargic as you begin your workout, then I would suggest drinking a small energy drink (*p.77*) and eating a banana half an hour before you start exercising.

After your workout, it is important that you replace the lost energy in the body's stores and refuel your metabolism at an optimum time: by putting carbohydrate energy back into the body immediately after you work out, you will actually elevate your metabolism for up to 10 hours after exercising. The ideal way of doing this is to eat a small amount of carbohydrate and protein within 15 minutes of finishing a workout, and then eating another small snack in the following half hour. I would suggest having a fruit smoothie, or a piece of fruit and some nuts when you finish your workout, and then a small bowl of cereal with yoghurt, or a low-fat snack bar containing seeds, half an hour later (*for other snack options, see p.44*).

Q Should I be feeling pain in my muscles to know that my workout has been effective?

a When you first start working out, your muscles can often feel slightly tight for a day or two afterwards. However, this feeling shouldn't present itself as a complete inability to move. This is where stretching is so important, since it relaxes and elongates the muscles to prevent stiffness and immobility (*pp.20–23*). Once you are working out

regularly, you should expect your muscles to feel as though they have been worked hard; if they don't, you may not be exercising effectively enough.

Q What are the ideal sports for me to do as a result of following the Endurance programme?

a I have designed the Endurance programme to be a total body workout that will give you improved performance in most sporting activities. The short blasts of aerobic activity in this PHA routine make it an ideal preparation for multi-sprint sports such as football and hockey. Also, the high average heart rate that you'll maintain during the whole workout makes it an excellent conditioning tool for endurance events such as rowing, running, cycling, and triathlon.

Q I've completed six weeks of the Bulking up programme and I want to start the Endurance workout. Can I combine the two?

a I would suggest that you stick to one programme or the other, not do both together. If you move from Bulking up to Endurance, you may notice a slight reduction in your muscle size, but your muscle strength will be relatively well-maintained on the Endurance plan.

153

endurance travel alternative

As with the main Endurance workout, the aim here is to perform all the exercises for a set period of time and then, as you become fitter, extend the amount of time that you perform each exercise.

Use the same timings as for the original workout, but for this travel alternative work your way right through the programme, and then repeat the sequence two more times in quick succession.

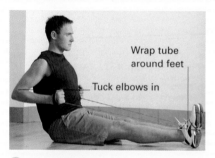

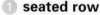

Wrap tube around feet

Tuck elbows in

2 jump squat, p.137

3 press-up, p.138

4 fixed lunge, p.139

5 advanced crunch, p.140

1 seated row

- Sit on the floor with legs straight
- Wrap exertube around feet until taut
- Pull handles into side of lower torso
- Return to start position
- Levels 1/2/3 = 30/45/60 secs

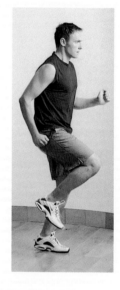

6 jogging on the spot

- Take short, fast steps on the spot
- Keep torso strong and upright
- Relax shoulders and neck
- Don't raise knees too high
- Breathe evenly
- Continue for 90 secs

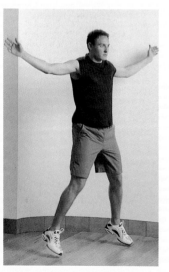

10 star jump

- Squat down with knees bent and back straight
- Exhale, leap up, and spread out arms and legs
- Inhale and return to squat position
- Levels 1/2/3 = 30/45/60 secs

11 advanced crossover, p.146

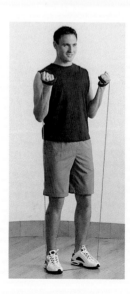

12 bicep curl

- Stand on the exertube, feet hip-width apart
- Wrap tube round hands until taut
- Face palms away from you
- Exhale and raise hands to shoulder height
- Inhale and lower hands to start position
- Levels 1/2/3 = 30/45/60 secs

key
1 see main workout
1 travel alternative

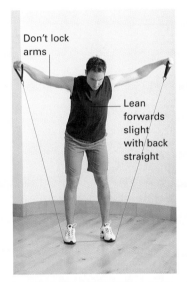

Don't lock arms

Lean forwards slight with back straight

7 reverse flye

- Stand on exertube, feet hip-width apart
- Grasp handles with palms facing inwards
- Exhale and raise arms out and away from sides
- Lift handles up to shoulder height
- Inhale and lower down to start position
- Levels 1/2/3 = 30/45/60 secs

8 seated squat, p.143

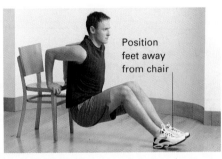

Position feet away from chair

9 tricep dip

- Hold chair seat, with palms facing backwards and arms extended
- Lower down until elbows are at 90°
- Push back up to start position
- Levels 1/2/3 = 30/45/60 secs

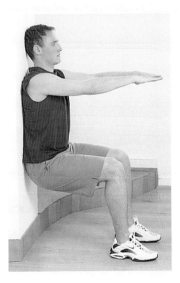

13 wall sit

- Lean against a wall
- Position feet a short distance from wall
- Inhale and lower torso until thighs are at 90° to floor
- Hold for 20–40 seconds, depending on fitness
- Exhale and push up to start position

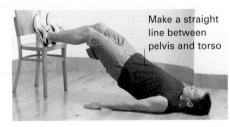

Make a straight line between pelvis and torso

14 body lift

- Lie on back on the floor, arms at sides
- Rest feet on chair and exhale
- Raise pelvis in a straight line with torso
- Inhale and lower to start position
- Levels 1/2/3 = 30/45/60 secs

15 reverse curl, p.151

endurance training log

As you notice yourself becoming fitter over the weeks, you should extend the amount of time that you perform each exercise before increasing the weights that you lift.

exercise	date: weight	time	date: weight	time	date: weight	time
pull-up set 1						
jump squat set 1						
press-up set 1						
fixed lunge set 1						
advanced crunch set 1						
pull-up set 2						
jump squat set 2						
press-up set 2						
fixed lunge set 2						
advanced crunch set 2						
rower or cross-trainer						
lateral pull-down set 1						
seated squat set 1						
tricep dip set 1						
bench step-up set 1						
advanced crossover set 1						

Even when you **feel fatigued**, keep **pushing** yourself **harder**

exercise (continued)	weight	time	weight	time	weight	time
lateral pull-down set 2						
seated squat set 2						
tricep dip set 2						
bench step-up set 2						
advanced crossover set 2						
rower or cross-trainer						
alternate bicep curl set 1						
leg extension set 1						
tricep push-down set 1						
hamstring curl set 1						
reverse curl set 1						
alternate bicep curl set 2						
leg extension set 2						
tricep push-down set 2						
hamstring curl set 2						
reverse curl set 2						
rower or cross-trainer						

choosing equipment

Whether you exercise at home on the Fat loss programme, or use the travel alternatives, all you need are a few well-chosen pieces of equipment.

Heart rate monitor
This is a really useful piece of kit. It consists of a band that you strap around your chest and a wrist watch (*see illustration, p.7*), and provides an instant and accurate display of your working heart rate while you exercise. Use it to increase or decrease the intensity of your workout so that you can achieve the maximum results.

The choice of heart rate monitors can be a little overwhelming, to say the least, but unless you are planning to take up sport seriously, you will not need to spend a fortune on this item. The most simple and cost-effective version will do. However, the most popular brand in the world is Polar. Other good brands are Nike, Suunto and Cyclosport.

Dumbbells
These are probably the most versatile pieces of equipment in terms of the range of exercises that you can perform with them. Invest in a couple of pairs of solid dumbbells in different weights with a comfortable grip. Popular brands are Golds, Kettler and York.

Exertube
Lengths of rubber tubing with handles at either end, exertubes may also be known as exercise bands or fit-tubes. They come in different strengths, so experiment with several before you buy to find one with a level of resistance that suits you best.

Fitness ball
A superb addition to any workout, fitness balls add an extra dimension to leg and ab workouts. They come in three sizes according to your height and weight. A medium-sized ball will suit most people.

useful addresses

Please note that, due to the fast-changing nature of the worldwide web, some websites may be out of date by the time you read this information.

In the UK and Republic of Ireland

matt roberts personal training
32–34 Jermyn Street
London SW1Y 6HS
Tel: 020 7439 8800
Email: info@personaltrainer.uk.com
www.personaltrainer.uk.com

Fitness Network
www.fitnessnetwork.co.uk

If equipment is not available in your local shops (particularly exertubes), try:
Physique Management
www.physique.uk.com

In Australia and New Zealand

Active for Life
www.activeforlife.com.au

Australian Fitness Network
Email: info@fitnessnetwork.com.au
www.fitnessnetwork.com.au

Healthinsite
www.healthinsite.gov.au

If equipment is not available in your local shops (particularly exertubes), try:
Fitness Works
www.fitnessworks.co.nz

Simple Fitness Solutions
www.simplefitnesssolutions.com

directory of exercises

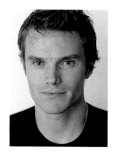

about the author

Matt Roberts, the UK's hottest personal trainer, began his career in fitness as an international sprinter. He went on to complete his studies at the American Council for Exercise and the American College of Sports Medicine. Known as "the personal trainer to the stars", Matt has a worldwide reputation for training celebrities, including Sandra Bullock, Trudie Styler, Mel C, Natalie Imbruglia, Naomi Campbell, Tom Ford, John Galliano, and Faye Dunaway.

Alongside his work with high-profile clients, he gets equal satisfaction from helping each person he trains to meet his or her health and fitness goals. And in his quest to make wellness accessible to everyone, he produces his own range of vitamins, home gym equipment, and body care products.

publisher's credits

The publisher would like to thank photographer John Davis and his assistants, John and V; Karen Mason for make-up and fantastic haircuts; Ruth Hope for styling; trainer Candy Outten; and models Louise Cole and Spencer Hayler from MOT, and Andrew Hingley and Caroline Wooten from Modelplan.

Special thanks to Nathan Burroughs and all the staff at Holmes Place, 80 Strand, London; King's Road Sporting Club, London, for lending the clothes; Helen and Anwar at The Village Studio, 101 Amies Street, London.

Finally, Dorling Kindersley would also like to thank Sara Robin for design assistance; Louise Waller for DTP assistance; Jennifer Lane and Shannon Beatty for editorial assistance; and Mark Cavanagh for the illustration on p.10.